THINK. LEAD. STAY.

Developing Respiratory Therapists Who Connect the Dots, Own Their Practice, and Build a Career Worth Keeping

PRETREVIS ELLISON REYNOLDS

Think. Lead. Stay.: Developing Respiratory Therapists Who Connect the Dots, Own Their Practice, and Build a Career Worth Keeping

This publication is intended for educational and informational purposes only. Although every effort has been made to ensure the accuracy of the information contained herein, the author makes no representations or warranties regarding the completeness, accuracy, or applicability of the content. Readers should use their professional judgment and follow the policies, procedures, and regulations of their employing institution, as well as applicable local, state, and federal laws.

The views and opinions expressed in this book are those of the author and do not necessarily reflect the views, policies, or positions of any employer, healthcare organization, professional association, or affiliated institution.

The clinical examples, scenarios, and conversations presented in this book are based on the author's professional experience. Identifying details have been changed, and in some cases composite characters and situations have been created to protect the privacy and confidentiality of patients, colleagues, and organizations. Any resemblance to actual persons or events is coincidental.

This book is not intended to replace formal education, institutional policies, clinical protocols, or professional medical judgment. Healthcare professionals should always follow the standards of practice and policies established by their employing organizations.

DEDICATION

In loving memory of my parents, John D & Carolyn Ellison.

Your love, sacrifices, and unwavering belief in me laid the foundation for every dream I've been blessed to pursue.

Though you are no longer here to hold this book in your hands, I carry your lessons, your strength, and your love with me every single day.

I hope I've made you proud.

TABLE OF CONTENTS

PREFACE

When I became a respiratory therapist, I thought success meant learning every procedure, memorizing every protocol, and mastering every ventilator.

Over time, I realized something was missing.

I watched bright, capable therapists complete orientation, pass competencies, and demonstrate technical proficiency, yet still hesitate when faced with a patient whose condition didn't match the textbook. They knew the steps, but they struggled to connect the dots.

As I transitioned into education, I began asking a different question.

What if orientation wasn't just about creating competent therapists? What if it was about developing critical thinkers?

That question changed everything.

This book grew from years of observing new graduates, experienced hires, preceptors, and leaders. It was shaped by conversations after difficult cases, debriefings following rapid responses, successes, mistakes, and countless moments where someone simply needed permission to think out loud.

Respiratory therapy is an incredible profession. We make life-changing decisions every day. But technical skill alone is no longer enough. Our profession needs clinicians who can analyze, adapt, communicate, teach, and lead.

That is the heart of this book.

Whether you're a new graduate beginning your career, a preceptor shaping the next generation, an educator designing orientation, or a leader building a stronger department, my hope is that these pages challenge you to think differently about professional development.

Because our goal shouldn't be to produce therapists who simply know what to do.

Our goal should be to develop professionals who understand **why**.

When that happens, they don't just become competent.

They become the kind of respiratory therapists who think, lead, and stay.

—Pretrevis Ellison Reynolds

ACKNOWLEDGMENTS

No meaningful journey is ever traveled alone, and this book is no exception.

First, I thank God for opening doors I never imagined and for continually reminding me that my purpose extends far beyond the bedside.

To my husband, **Jamal,** thank you for loving me so well. You have never questioned my dreams; you only asked how you could help make them happen. And whenever an obstacle appeared, your response was always the same: "We'll figure it out." Those words have given me courage more times than you know. Every milestone I've reached since we've met has been sweeter because you've been there to celebrate it, and every challenge has felt lighter because you've carried it with me. Thank you for being my partner and one of God's greatest blessings in my life.

To my sons, **Quin, RJ, and Raelon,** thank you for giving my life its greatest purpose. Every goal I've pursued, every challenge I've accepted, and every dream I've chased has been fueled by my desire to show you what is possible through faith, perseverance, and hard work. I hope my journey has taught you that it is never too late to pursue your dreams, that setbacks do not define you, and that excellence is built one intentional step at a time. You have always been, and will always be, my greatest "why." I love each of you more than words could ever express, and I couldn't be prouder of the men you have become.

To my sisters, thank you for being part of my journey in your own unique ways. And to my youngest sister, **Isheka**, thank you for always being in my corner. Your love and encouragement have meant more than you'll ever know.

To my forever best friend, **Lissa**, thank you for standing beside me through every season of life. Thank you for your loyalty, your encouragement, and for being the kind of friend who has felt more like family since childhood. Life has been better because you've been in it.

To my mentor, **Dr. Gregory Evans,** thank you for seeing potential in me long before I fully saw it in myself. You challenged me to think bigger, pushed me beyond the comfort of the bedside, and encouraged me to pursue opportunities I never imagined possible. Your mentorship, encouragement, and unwavering belief in my abilities have shaped not only my career, but the leader and person I have become. Thank you for continually asking, **"Why not you?"** Those three words challenged me to dream bigger, lead boldly, and believe that I belonged in every room where I could make a difference. I will always be grateful for the time, wisdom, and confidence you poured into me.

To my amazing best friends who are also respiratory therapists—**Jasmine, Vester, Nicole, Tomeka, Felicia, Dominique, and Kristi**—thank you for walking this journey with me. Thank you for the laughter, the lessons learned through challenges, and the friendships that only God could have orchestrated. You have each shaped not only the professional I have become, but the person I am today.

Finally, to every respiratory therapist, student, preceptor, educator, and leader who chooses to invest in others: this book is for you. May you continue to ask questions, challenge assumptions, encourage growth, and never stop connecting the dots.

To **Ryan**, thank you for believing in me, trusting my vision, and creating the space for me to grow as a leader and educator.

Together, we will build the future of respiratory care.

INTRODUCTION

Why I Almost Didn't Write This Book

"Sometimes the thing you were meant to do finds you, usually when you are busy trying to walk away from it."

The List

It started with a phone call from a friend.

I was working as a clinical liaison at a rehabilitation facility, deliberately, intentionally far from the ICU, far from ventilators, far from the kind of high-stakes clinical environment I had given twenty years of my life to. I had made a quiet decision that most people around me didn't fully understand, and that I hadn't fully explained, because explaining it would have required admitting something I wasn't quite ready to say out loud.

I was done. Not retired. I was still working, still showing up, still functioning. But something essential had gone quiet inside me, the way a room goes quiet after everyone leaves. I was present in body and absent in spirit, and I had made a kind of peace with that. I told myself I was resting. I told myself I was transitioning. What I was actually doing was surviving one day at a time, in a role that asked very little of my heart, which was exactly what I needed because my heart had very little left to give.

COVID had seen to that.

I won't spend pages describing what the pandemic did to respiratory therapists, because if you are reading this book, you already know. You lived some version of it yourself. You know what it looks like to watch colleagues break under the weight of impossible circumstances. You know the particular exhaustion that comes not only from the physical demands of the work but also from the grief it carries: the accumulated, unprocessed grief of loss after loss after loss, in rooms where families couldn't visit, patients struggled to breathe, and respiratory therapists stood at the center of it all, doing everything they could. Sometimes it was enough. Sometimes it wasn't.

I was burned out. I was grieving. I was numb in the specific way that people become numb when feeling everything has become too costly. I was all of those things at once, and I had done what many clinicians do when they reach that point: I had found a quieter corner of the healthcare world and had settled into it, grateful for the distance.

And then my friend called.

Why Not You?

She worked at a hospital with an open position: a hospital-based clinical educator in the respiratory care department. She wasn't calling to offer it to me. She was calling because she knew I knew people, and she needed a recommendation.

I carefully went through my mental list. I thought about the colleagues I had worked alongside over two decades across ICUs, emergency departments, NICUs, and LTACs in hospitals across multiple states during my years as a travel therapist. I thought about who had the clinical depth, the communication skills, the patience, the genuine investment in developing other people that a role like this required.

I came up with a name. My friend agreed she was a strong candidate. We hung up feeling good about the solution.

Except the candidate decided the timing wasn't right for her.

So, my friend called again. We went back to the drawing board together, talking through options, weighing names. And then, in the middle of that conversation, she asked me a question that stopped me completely.

"Why not you?"

My first instinct was resistance: immediate, reflexive, almost indignant resistance, the kind that rises up when someone suggests something that threatens the careful equilibrium you have constructed around your own limitations. I had reasons. Good ones, I thought. I was settled where I was. I wasn't sure I had anything left to pour into a role that demanding. I had spent twenty years accumulating clinical experience and leadership wisdom, and I wasn't convinced any of it was still accessible to me, buried as it was under everything COVID had deposited on top of it.

I said something noncommittal, and we ended the call.

And then I sat with it.

That night, and the nights that followed, I had the kind of quiet internal conversation that only happens when a question has gotten under your skin far enough that ignoring it requires more energy than answering it. I called close friends, people who had known me across the long arc of my career, who had worked beside me, watched me lead, and seen me at my best and worst. I wasn't looking for cheerleading. I was looking for truth.

What they gave me was both.

They reminded me, with the particular directness that real friends are capable of, that I had been doing this work for years without a title. That I was the colleague people came to when they were confused about a patient and afraid to ask anyone official. That I was the one who stayed after a difficult shift to debrief with a newer RT who needed to process what had happened. That I had been leading quietly, from the side, building people up in the margins of a role that never formally asked me to, because I couldn't help it, because it was simply who I was, because the development of other respiratory therapists was woven into me so deeply that I had been doing it accidentally for my entire career.

"You have a lot to offer," they said. "More than you can see right now."

I had heard something like that before, years earlier, from a medical director in an ICU, who had seen leadership potential in me long before I recognized it in myself. He had given me responsibility before I felt ready for it, included me in conversations above my pay grade, and trusted me with things that quietly expanded my sense of what was possible for me in this profession. I had spent the years since trying to become, for others, what he had been for me.

Maybe, I thought, this was the role where I could finally do that with intention.

I hesitantly applied.

What I Found on the Other Side

The first weeks in the educator role were, to put it generously, humbling.

Not because I lacked clinical knowledge (twenty years across every RT setting imaginable had given me plenty of that). But because walking into a department as its educator meant seeing, with sudden and uncomfortable clarity, everything the existing system was not doing for the people inside it. The gaps in orientation. The preceptors doing their absolute best with no preparation for the teaching part of precepting. The new RTs who were technically cleared for independent practice but emotionally nowhere near ready for what it actually felt like. The quiet, slow erosion of engagement in staff who had stopped being asked what they needed or where they wanted to go.

I had seen versions of this before as a traveler moving through different hospital systems, as a supervisor and manager watching staff from a different vantage point, as the colleague who had tried to step in informally when a new RT was being failed by a neglectful preceptor, knowing it wasn't my place but unable to do nothing. I had always known the problem existed. Now I had the role and the responsibility to actually do something about it.

The exhaustion didn't disappear overnight. The grief didn't either. But something else began to happen, something I had stopped expecting.

I started to feel energized.

Not the brittle, adrenaline-fueled energy of a busy clinical shift, but something slower and more sustaining. The energy that comes from work that is aligned with your deepest purpose. I would leave a conversation with a new RT (one where something had clicked for them, where I had watched understanding move across their face like light coming through a window) and I would feel, for the first time in a long time, like I was exactly where I was supposed to be.

And then one day, I watched a new RT handle a complex patient situation with a confidence and a clinical reasoning process that I recognized. Not because it was textbook, but because it was something we had talked through together. Something I had intentionally put in place. A framework I had given them, not just a task I had taught them to perform.

They didn't need me in the room. They had internalized the thinking.

That was the moment. That was when I knew, without any doubt, without any of the hesitation that had followed me into this role, that this was exactly where I was supposed to be.

And this book is what happened next.

What This Book Is and Who It's For

Think. Lead. Stay. is the book I wish had existed when I was trying to figure out how to do this work well. It is the book I would have handed to every preceptor I ever watched struggle in silence, every educator I ever met who was doing their best with no roadmap, every department leader who genuinely wanted to develop their staff and didn't know where to begin.

It is not a textbook. It will not ask you to memorize frameworks or pass a test at the end of the chapter. It is a conversation, the kind that happens between colleagues who trust each other enough to be honest about the gap between what respiratory therapy education currently does and what it could do if we invested in it with the same rigor and intention we bring to clinical competency.

The book is built around three pillars that I have come to believe are the foundation of everything we are trying to build:

Think, because clinical judgment cannot be checked off a competency form, and developing respiratory therapists who reason through complexity rather than just respond to it is the most important clinical education work we can do.

Lead, because leadership is not a title, and every RT in your department is already leading in some way, whether you have named it or not. Our job is to develop that capacity intentionally, at every level, starting with the people who teach new RTs how to think: the preceptors.

Stay, because retention is not a perk problem or a scheduling problem or a compensation problem at its core. It is a development problem. People stay where they are growing, where they are seen, where they belong. Building that kind of department is the most important leadership work any educator can do.

Each section of this book addresses one of these pillars (what it means, why it matters, and what you can do about it) starting Monday. Not in an ideal department with an unlimited budget and administrative buy-in at every level. In your actual department, with your actual constraints, with the people and the time and the resources you actually have.

Because that is where the work happens. Not in theory. In the real world, on the real floor, in the real moments that shape whether a new RT becomes the clinician they are capable of becoming or quietly becomes a statistic in the next workforce turnover report.

A Note About the Stories in This Book

The patients, colleagues, and new RTs who appear in these pages are real in the sense that every story is drawn from real experience accumulated over twenty years of clinical practice, leadership, travel therapy, precepting, supervising, and educating. Names and identifying details have been changed to protect privacy. In some cases, composite characters represent patterns I have witnessed across multiple people and settings rather than a single individual.

What has not been changed is the truth of what happened, what it felt like, and what it taught me. These are honest stories from an honest career, including the parts where I got it wrong, where I didn't yet have the tools, where I watched something unfold that I couldn't stop and carried the weight of that longer than I should have.

I am telling you these things because I want you to trust me. And trust, in my experience, is built not on credentials but on honesty. I have the credentials (the years, the certifications, the roles, the MBA I finished last weekend while raising three young men, settling into a new marriage, and running a consulting business) because, apparently, I have never met a challenge I didn't immediately decide to take on simultaneously with three others. But credentials tell you what I know. Stories tell you who I am.

I hope, by the end of this book, you feel like you know me. And I hope that knowing me makes it easier to do the brave, important, often underappreciated work of developing the next generation of respiratory therapists.

They need you. More than they know how to say. More than the system has taught them to ask for.

This book is for them and for you. Let's begin.

How to Use This Book

Think. Lead. Stay. is organized into five parts, moving from problem to solution to practice. You can read it straight through, or you can go directly to the section most relevant to where you are right now. Each chapter ends with reflection prompts that work equally well for individual journaling or group discussion; they make excellent starting points for a Preceptor Power Hour, a staff development session, or a leadership team conversation.

If you are a clinical educator: this entire book is for you, but Parts Two through Five are where you will find the most immediately actionable material.

If you are a preceptor: Chapter Two and Chapter Eight were written with you specifically in mind. Start there if you need to.

If you are a department leader or manager: Part Four (Stay) addresses the retention and culture questions that keep most leaders up at night. You might start there and work backward.

And if you are a new RT who somehow found this book: Chapter Fifteen is a letter written directly to you. Go read it first. Then come back and read the rest, because understanding what your educators and preceptors are trying to build for you will make you a better partner in your own development.

Wherever you start, welcome. I am glad you are here.

And I am especially glad that my friend wouldn't take no for an answer.

"Sometimes the thing you were meant to do finds you, usually when you are busy trying to walk away from it."

01

ORIENTATION IS NOT EDUCATION

"We are what we repeatedly do. Excellence, then, is not an act but a habit." – (Will Durant) summarizing Aristotle (which feels appropriate, since we have been summarizing other people's work and calling it orientation for years.)

The Signature That Changed How I See Everything

I want to tell you about a competency form.

Not because competency forms are inherently villainous. They are not. They serve a purpose, and that purpose matters. But this particular form, on this particular afternoon, became the moment that crystallized everything I had been quietly sensing about the gap between what we call orientation and what orientation actually does.

I was reviewing documentation, the kind of administrative task that sounds mundane until you find something in it that stops you cold, when I came across a completed competency checklist for a relatively new respiratory therapist. Every box was checked. Every skill had been observed and verified. The signatures were all in the right places. On paper, this RT was ready. Competent. Cleared for independent practice.

I had been in a patient room with this same RT two days earlier.

We were at the bedside of a patient whose condition was changing, subtly but unmistakably. The kind of change that experienced eyes catch early and inexperienced eyes miss entirely, not because they aren't looking, but because they don't yet know what they're looking for. I watched this RT complete every task correctly. Vitals checked. Settings verified. Documentation accurate. Then I asked, as casually as I could manage, "What are you thinking about this patient right now?"

The pause that followed was long enough to be its own answer.

"I'm thinking... everything looks okay?" they said, with the particular upward inflection of someone who was hoping they had given the right answer rather than someone who actually believed it.

Everything did not look okay. And this RT, through absolutely no fault of their own, lacked the clinical reasoning framework to see why. They had been taught to look. They had not been taught to see.

And yet the competency form said "ready."

I put the form down, stared at the ceiling for a moment, and wondered how many versions of this scenario were playing out across respiratory therapy departments every single day. New RTs completing orientations, receiving signed forms, and stepping into independent practice carrying a gap so significant it was practically load-bearing, a gap not in their knowledge of what to do, but in their understanding of why.

That is the problem this chapter is about. And it is bigger, more systemic, and more solvable than most departments realize.

Let's Talk About What Orientation Actually Is

Orientation, in most respiratory therapy departments, is a beautifully organized list of things a new RT needs to be able to do.

Complete a ventilator check. Administer a breathing treatment. Perform an arterial blood gas. Set up CPAP. Assist with intubation. Document in the electronic health record. Know where the code cart is. Complete the mandatory modules (yes, all twelve of them, including the one about fire safety that everyone clicks through at approximately the speed of light).

There is nothing wrong with any of this. These are real skills. They matter. A new RT who cannot perform them competently is a patient safety concern, and orientation exists precisely to address that.

But here is the question I want you to sit with: What happens when the patient doesn't follow the checklist?

Because patients, as any experienced clinician will tell you with a tired smile, are remarkably inconsistent about following the checklist. They deteriorate in ways the protocol didn't anticipate. They present with comorbidities that complicate the straightforward intervention. They are anxious, or noncompliant, or physiologically unusual, or all three simultaneously at three in the morning, when the supervising physician is unavailable and the new RT is standing at the bedside with a perfectly signed competency form and no idea what to do next.

This is the moment orientation prepares new RTs to perform. It is not, in most departments, the moment orientation prepares them to think through.

And that distinction, between performance and reasoning, between task completion and clinical judgment, is the difference between a competent RT and a capable one. Between an RT who can function when everything goes according to plan and one who can navigate when it doesn't.

The Competency Illusion

Let me introduce you to a concept I call the Competency Illusion, which is my way of describing what happens when a signed checklist becomes a proxy for genuine readiness.

The Competency Illusion works like this: we design a list of observable skills, we watch someone perform those skills under supervised conditions, and when they perform them correctly, we conclude that they are prepared. The form gets signed. The orientation period ends. The new RT transitions to independent practice. Everyone breathes a small sigh of relief and moves on.

What the signed form cannot tell us (and no signed form can) is whether the RT understands the clinical reasoning behind what they just demonstrated. Whether they could recognize when the standard approach isn't working. Whether they know what question to ask when something feels off but they can't yet name why. Whether they have the judgment, under pressure, to prioritize competing demands and make the call that best serves the patient.

These things are not captured on a checklist. They are developed over time, through deliberate reflection and guided experience, by educators and preceptors who understand that their job is not just to observe task performance but to cultivate clinical thinking.

The problem is that competency checklists are efficient, documentable, and legally defensible. Clinical reasoning development is slower, messier, harder to quantify, and requires a level of investment that many departments, understaffed, under-resourced, and under pressure, struggle to sustain. So we default to the checklist. We sign the form. And we call it orientation.

To be clear: I am not suggesting we abandon competency verification. Please do not abandon competency verification. A respiratory therapist who cannot correctly set up a ventilator circuit is a problem that a competency checklist exists to catch, and that matters enormously. What I am suggesting is that the checklist is the floor, and we have been treating it as the ceiling.

What New RTs Are Actually Walking Into

Let me paint you a picture of a typical first solo shift for a new respiratory therapist who has just completed orientation.

They arrive early because new RTs always do, partly out of professionalism and partly because they need the extra fifteen minutes to find everything and remember where the bathroom is. They receive their assignment. They review their patients. They feel, simultaneously, a surge of pride at being here, a flutter of excitement at doing this for real, and a low-grade terror, completely appropriate given the circumstances, that nobody warned them would last approximately eighteen months.

They walk into their first patient room alone.

The patient is not the patient from the simulation. The patient is a seventy-three-year-old with COPD, heart failure, and a personality that can most charitably be described as "spirited." The ventilator settings are within parameters, but something about the waveforms looks slightly different from what the new RT is used to seeing. Is it different enough to matter? They are not sure. They complete the assessment. They document. They move on, because the assignment is full and there is no time to stand at a bedside wondering, and also because they don't want anyone to think they don't know what they're doing.

At the end of the shift, they go home. They are exhausted. They replay moments from the day in their head with the obsessive detail that only new clinicians and people who have said the wrong thing at a dinner party truly understand. They wonder if they missed something. They probably didn't. But they don't know how to know.

This is the reality of what we send new RTs into when orientation ends. Not a controlled environment with a preceptor nearby. The real floor, with real patients, with the full weight of independent practice, often far sooner than any of them feel ready for it.

And we are surprised when some of them struggle.

The 12-Month Cliff (and Why It Is Entirely Predictable)

Here is a pattern I have watched repeat itself across departments, hospital systems, and states, with a consistency that stopped surprising me a long time ago.

A new RT completes orientation. They spend the next several months in a kind of managed survival mode, learning the rhythms of the department, building relationships with colleagues, developing the procedural fluency that comes only from repetition. They are working hard. They are growing. From the outside, things look fine.

Then, somewhere around the twelve-to-eighteen-month mark, something shifts.

For some RTs, it is the moment they realize they are competent enough to recognize how much they still don't know, and that the formal support that helped them through orientation is long gone. For others, it is the point at which the initial excitement of a new career has settled into the reality of the daily work, and the question, "Is this where I want to be?" starts to surface. For others still, it is simply that they have developed enough confidence to start looking around at other departments, other specialties, other opportunities, and what they see elsewhere looks more appealing than what they have been given where they are.

This is the 12-Month Cliff. And it is not a mystery. It is not a generational quirk or a sign that new RTs lack commitment. It is a predictable consequence of a system that invests heavily in getting people through the door and very little in what happens after they arrive.

The departments that retain their RTs past that cliff are not doing something magical. They are doing something intentional. They have recognized that orientation is the beginning of development, not its end, and have built structures, relationships, and cultures that reflect that understanding.

The good news is that those structures are buildable. In any department. With any budget. By any educator who is willing to see their role as something bigger than orientation logistics.

That is what the rest of this book is about.

What Education Actually Looks Like

If orientation is the floor, education is everything built on top of it. And education, in the context of developing respiratory therapists, looks less like a classroom and more like a series of intentional relationships and structured experiences that happen over time, in the actual clinical environment, with real patients and real stakes.

It looks like a preceptor who narrates their clinical reasoning out loud instead of just demonstrating the skill. "Before I make this change, I'm asking myself, what does this waveform tell me about what this patient's lungs are doing right now?"

It looks like an educator who sits down with a new RT after a complex case and asks, not "Did you do everything correctly?" but "Walk me through what you were thinking. What did you notice first? What did you consider? What would you do differently?"

It looks like a department culture where not knowing something is an invitation to learn rather than an occasion for embarrassment. Where the new RT who says "I'm not sure, can you help me think through this?" is celebrated rather than quietly judged.

It looks like a thirty-sixty-ninety-day development plan that continues long after the competency forms are signed, not because the RT isn't ready, but because readiness is not a destination. It is an ongoing process that never really ends, for any of us, at any stage of our careers.

Education, in other words, is orientation with a longer time horizon and a deeper purpose. It is the difference between preparing someone to perform and preparing someone to grow. And growing respiratory therapists, ones who think critically, lead confidently, and stay because they are genuinely invested, is the most important work any of us in this profession will ever do.

A Word to the Skeptic

I recognize that somewhere in this chapter, a reader has been nodding along with one part of their brain while another part is running a quiet counter-argument that sounds something like: "This is all well and good, but I work in a department with three open positions, mandatory overtime, and a manager who thinks education is whatever happens during the annual competency fair. What exactly am I supposed to do with this?"

First of all, I see you. I have been you. That reality is real, and it is hard, and it deserves to be named rather than papered over with optimistic frameworks.

Second, the tools in this book are specifically designed for the real world, not the ideal one. They do not require a dedicated simulation center, a full-time education budget, or an administration that has already bought in. Most of them require nothing more than a willing educator, fifteen minutes, and the decision to do one thing differently starting Monday.

You cannot build everything at once. You can build something. And something, done consistently and with intention, has a way of becoming everything, slowly, and then all at once. That is how cultures change. Not with grand gestures, but with the accumulation of small, intentional acts that eventually become the way things are done around here.

So start small. Start Monday. And keep reading, because the rest of this book is full of exactly what you need to begin.

Chapter Summary

- Orientation and education are not the same thing. Orientation prepares new RTs to perform skills under known conditions. Education develops the clinical reasoning, judgment, and professional identity that allow them to thrive when conditions change, which they always do.

- The Competency Illusion occurs when signed checklists are treated as evidence of full readiness. Competency verification is necessary and important, but it is the floor, not the ceiling, of what new RT development should accomplish.

- The 12-Month Cliff (the predictable spike in turnover that occurs between twelve and eighteen months) is not a mystery. It is a direct consequence of systems that invest in orientation and then stop. It is preventable with intentional, ongoing development structures.

- Education in the clinical setting looks like narrated reasoning, reflective debriefing, psychological safety, and a culture that treats growth as a continuous process rather than a box to check.

- You do not need a perfect department or an unlimited budget to begin. You need intention, consistency, and the willingness to do one thing differently starting Monday.

Reflection Prompts

1. Think about your department's current orientation process. Where does it excel at building clinical skill? Where does it fall short in building clinical thinking? What is one specific gap you could begin to address?

2. Have you ever signed a competency form for someone you weren't fully confident was ready, because the timeline demanded it, or because there was no other option? What did that moment feel like, and what did it tell you about the system?

3. Who in your department is currently approaching the 12-Month Cliff? What do they need from you before they get there?

4. If you could add one thing to your orientation process that focused specifically on clinical reasoning rather than task performance, what would it be?

Coming Up in Chapter Two

We have named the limits of orientation and introduced the gap that exists between competency and capability. In Chapter Two, we turn to one of the most significant and most overlooked contributors to that gap: the preceptor relationship. Because how new RTs are taught matters just as much as what they are taught. And in most departments, the people doing the teaching have never been taught how to teach.

That is where we are going next.

"The competency form is the floor.
Education is everything built on top of it."

02

THE PRECEPTOR PROBLEM

"The best teachers are those who show you where to look but don't tell you what to see."
– Alexandra K. Trenfor

The Day I Realized I Wasn't as Good at This as I Thought

I remember her name, but I'll call her Maya.

She was a new graduate, bright, eager, and the kind of orientee who showed up early, stayed late, and asked questions that made you think she would be exceptional. She had strong fundamentals. Her assessment skills were solid. On paper, she was doing everything right.

I was her preceptor.

And I was, by every external measure, an experienced respiratory therapist. I had years of clinical practice behind me. I had worked in the ICU, the ED, and the NICU. I had managed complex ventilator patients, run codes, and navigated the kind of high-stakes moments that make newer clinicians freeze. I knew my craft. I was confident. I was ready to pass that knowledge on.

What I didn't realize, not yet, was that knowing your craft and being able to teach it are two completely different skills. And no one had ever taught me the difference.

About three weeks into Maya's orientation, I noticed something. She was quieter than usual during patient rounds. She completed her tasks efficiently, charted on time, and followed protocols correctly. But when I asked her what she was thinking, really thinking, about a patient who was beginning to decompensate, she looked at me with something I will never forget. It wasn't confusion. It was something closer to fear. Not of the patient, but of getting the answer wrong in front of me.

That look stopped me cold.

I had been so focused on showing her what to do that I had never once invited her into how I was thinking. I had been performing competence in front of her instead of teaching it. I was so comfortable in my own clinical reasoning that I had forgotten it was ever uncomfortable. As a result, I had left her alone with her uncertainty instead of walking through it with her.

I was a great clinician. I was a mediocre preceptor.

The hardest part of that realization wasn't the humility it required. I came to understand that Maya wasn't struggling because she wasn't capable. She was struggling because I wasn't equipped. And if I, someone who genuinely cared, who showed up, who wanted her to succeed, could miss that so completely, what was happening in preceptor relationships where the investment was even less intentional?

That question changed everything about how I approached education.

This chapter is about that gap, the space between clinical excellence and teaching excellence, and why closing it is one of the most important things our profession can do.

The Assumption That's Costing Us

There is an assumption quietly embedded in how respiratory therapy departments operate across the country, and it goes something like this:

If someone is a strong clinician, they will be a strong preceptor.

It sounds reasonable. It feels intuitive. Yet it is almost entirely wrong.

Think about what we actually do when we assign a preceptor. We look for experience. We look for clinical competence. We look for someone who shows up consistently and knows what they're doing. Those are reasonable criteria, but they work for identifying a skilled therapist, not a skilled teacher. And we are asking them to do something entirely different: take the complex, often unconscious web of knowledge and judgment they have spent years building, and make it visible, accessible, and transferable to someone who is just beginning.

That is a skill. A learnable, developable, absolutely-not-automatic skill.

And yet, in most departments, here is what preceptor preparation looks like: a brief conversation with a charge therapist or manager, perhaps a form to fill out, and then, orientation begins. The new RT shows up on Monday morning, and the preceptor is expected to know how to guide, teach, give feedback, manage a patient load, read the learner's emotional state, calibrate when to step in and when to let the learner struggle productively, and build a trusting relationship, all at the same time.

We would never hand a new RT a ventilator and say, "You'll figure it out." But we do something remarkably similar to our preceptors every single day.

The result is not that preceptors fail. Most do their absolute best with what they have been given. The result is that new RTs experience wildly inconsistent orientations that have more to do with who they are assigned to than what their department has intentionally built. And that inconsistency has consequences that ripple out for years.

Three Preceptors You've Already Met

In over twenty years of working in respiratory therapy as a clinician, a traveler, a manager, a preceptor, and now as a hospital-based clinical educator, I have had the privilege, and sometimes the frustration, of seeing preceptor relationships up close from every angle. I have been the orientee. I have been the preceptor. I have supervised preceptors. I have sat with new RTs in quiet hallways and listened to what they were actually experiencing.

What I have found is that most preceptors, regardless of the department or hospital system, tend to fall into one of three patterns. You will likely recognize all three immediately, because you have either had one, been one, or worked alongside one.

The Sink-or-Swimmer

"I learned the hard way. So will you."

This preceptor is not cruel. Let me be clear about that. In most cases, they are not even aware of what they are doing. They genuinely believe that struggle is the best teacher, and in some ways, they are not entirely wrong. Productive struggle is an important part of learning. But there is a profound difference between struggle that builds and struggle that breaks, and the Sink-or-Swimmer has not learned to tell the difference.

This preceptor learned through trial and error, in high-stakes situations where they had no choice but to figure it out, and in a culture that valued toughness over support. And because they survived that, because they emerged as a capable clinician, they have unconsciously concluded that the process that shaped them is the process that shapes everyone.

What the new RT experiences with this preceptor is a kind of loneliness disguised as independence. They are given tasks. They are evaluated on whether the tasks are completed correctly. But the space between "here is what to do" and "here is how to think about what to do" is never crossed. The orientee finishes their shift either having gotten through it or not, and either way, the why behind the clinical decisions remains a mystery.

The new RT trained by a Sink-or-Swimmer may become technically competent. They may even become a Sink-or-Swimmer themselves one day, because it is the only model of precepting they have ever seen. But they rarely become confident clinical thinkers. And they almost always remember the feeling of being alone in a room with a patient they weren't sure how to help, with no one to think out loud with.

The Protector

"Just do it my way and you'll be fine."

This preceptor loves their orientees. That is the first thing you need to understand about them. They are warm and reassuring, and new RTs often feel genuinely safe with them, which makes this pattern particularly difficult to identify as a problem.

The Protector's instinct is to smooth every rough edge, answer every question before the learner has a chance to sit with it, and step in the moment something becomes uncertain. Their intentions are beautiful. Their impact, over time, is quietly limiting.

What the Protector does not realize is that by removing difficulty, they are also removing the very experiences a new RT needs in order to develop clinical judgment. Judgment does not develop in comfort. It develops at the edge of what you know, when you are asked to reason your way through something unfamiliar. Every time the Protector steps in a moment too soon, they are borrowing against the new RT's future confidence without either of them realizing it.

The orientee with a Protector often thrives during orientation and struggles when it ends. Because during orientation, there was always someone there to catch them. And on the first shift they work alone, they realize with sudden clarity that the safety net was the preceptor, not their own developing judgment.

This is not a failure of the new RT. It is a failure of the model.

The Developer

"Tell me what you're thinking before we walk in."

This is the preceptor we are trying to build.

The Developer is not necessarily the most clinically gifted therapist in the department. They may not have the most years of experience. What they have is an understanding, whether intuitive or learned, that their job is not to demonstrate competence. Their job is to cultivate it.

The Developer asks questions before giving answers. They narrate their own thinking out loud so the learner can see inside a clinical mind at work. They let the new RT struggle for a moment, not cruelly, but purposefully, and then they debrief that struggle in a way that turns it into a lesson rather than a wound. They pay attention to the emotional state of their orientee, not just their task completion. They know the difference between a learner who needs more information and a learner who needs more confidence.

When a Developer preceptor finishes an orientation, the new RT doesn't just know the protocols. They know how to think. And that knowledge belongs to them; it doesn't walk out the door when the preceptor does.

Here is the important truth about Developers: very few of them were born. Most of them were made. They were made because someone invested in them, gave them language for what they were doing, and created space for them to reflect on their practice as educators, not just as clinicians.

That is exactly what Preceptor Power Hours are designed to do. And we will get to that. But first, we need to talk about what the research, and frankly, what the hallway conversations, tell us about what new RTs actually experience.

What New RTs Are Really Telling Us

I want to share something that I have collected over years of sitting with students and new RTs in the in-between moments. Not in formal evaluations, not in preceptor feedback forms, but in the honest, unguarded conversations that happen when someone finally feels safe enough to tell you the truth.

Here is what they say, over and over again, in different words, in different hospitals, and in different states:

"I didn't want to ask because I didn't want to seem stupid."

"I could tell my preceptor was annoyed when I asked questions."

"I knew what I was supposed to do. I just didn't know why."

"I felt like I was being tested, not taught."

"There were days I went home and cried, wondering if I had made the right choice."

"The one preceptor who changed everything for me simply asked me what I was thinking. Nobody had ever done that before."

Read those again.

Slowly.

These are not complaints from weak or uncommitted new graduates. They are the honest experiences of intelligent, capable people navigating one of the most vulnerable transitions of their professional lives, from student to therapist, often without the guidance they needed. And the thread running through all of them is not a lack of clinical content. It is a lack of connection. A lack of someone willing to sit in the uncertainty with them rather than just showing them how to get through it.

This is the preceptor problem. And it is ours to solve.

The Cost We Stop Counting

Let me be direct about what happens when we don't address this.

New RTs who experience unsupportive or underprepared preceptor relationships are significantly more likely to leave the profession within the first two years. They are more likely to experience burnout and compassion fatigue early in their careers. They are more likely to develop what I call clinical anxiety: a pattern of second-guessing and self-doubt that persists long after the clinical knowledge has settled, because the environment in which they learned did not feel safe enough to make mistakes and grow from them.

And here is the part that breaks my heart a little every time I think about it: we lose some of the best ones. Not the ones who couldn't handle it. The ones who cared too much to remain in a system that didn't invest in them. The ones who had every quality we need in the next generation of RT educators and leaders, and who left because nobody showed them what was possible.

That loss is more than a workforce problem. It is a patient care problem. It is a professional identity problem. And it is a solvable problem if we are willing to take preceptor development as seriously as we take clinical competency.

What This Chapter Is Asking of You

If you are reading this as a clinical educator, I want to ask you something gently but directly: How are your preceptors being prepared right now? Not evaluated. Prepared. What do they know about teaching clinical judgment? What tools do they have for giving feedback that builds rather than deflates? What space exists for them to talk honestly about the difficult parts of precepting: the orientee who is struggling, the shift that went sideways, the moment they weren't sure what to do?

If you are reading this as a preceptor, I want to say something that I needed to hear twenty years ago: the fact that you care about your orientee's success already puts you ahead of where I was. Caring is the foundation. But caring alone is not enough, and that is not your fault. It is a system failure. You were handed a role without a roadmap, and you have been doing your best with what you have. This book is the roadmap.

And if you are reading this as a new RT who is quietly recognizing their own orientation in these pages, in the loneliness, the uncertainty, and the moments of wondering if you were the only one who felt this way, I want you to know something: you were not alone. You were never alone. You were just in a system that hadn't yet figured out how to walk beside you properly.

That is what we are here to change.

Chapter Summary

- Being a great clinician does not automatically make someone a great preceptor. These are two distinct skill sets, and treating them as the same is costing us new RTs, experienced preceptors, and ultimately our patients.
- Most preceptors fall into one of three patterns: the Sink-or-Swimmer, the Protector, and the Developer. The goal is not to judge which pattern a preceptor currently occupies, but to understand what each pattern produces and intentionally develop more Developers.
- New RTs consistently report feeling alone, afraid to ask questions, and unsure of the why behind

clinical decisions. These are not personal failures. They are systemic ones.

- The cost of underprepared preceptors is measured in early burnout, early departure, and lost potential for the RT, for the department, and for patients.
- Preceptor development is not a luxury or an add-on. It is a core function of a healthy respiratory care department.

Reflection Prompts

Take a few minutes to reflect on these questions. If you are using this book as part of a team development process, these make excellent discussion starters for a Preceptor Power Hour.

1. Think back to your own orientation as a new RT. Which of the three preceptor types did you experience? What did that teach you about clinical practice, and about how you wanted, or didn't want, to show up for others?
2. If you have served as a preceptor, which pattern do you think you most naturally fall into? What would it take to move more consistently toward the Developer?
3. What is one thing your preceptors currently do not have, whether in preparation, tools, or support that you could begin to address this month?
4. Think of a new RT who struggled during orientation. Looking back, how much of that

struggle was about the learner, and how much was about the environment and the support they received?

Coming Up in Chapter Three

We have named the problem and looked honestly at what new RTs experience during the preceptor relationship. In Chapter Three, we turn to the longer arc: why good RTs leave, what the data tells us, and what conversations in hospital hallways reveal that exit interviews never capture. Because understanding why people leave is the first step toward building something worth staying for.

"*The best preceptors are not the ones who had all the answers. They are the ones who made it safe not to have them yet.*"

03

WHY GOOD RTs LEAVE

"People don't leave jobs. They leave environments where they stopped mattering."
– Unknown

The Night I Almost Became a Statistic

There was a night I remember clearly, because nights like that tend to stay with you, when I sat in my car in a hospital parking garage and asked myself a question I never expected to ask.

Is this still worth it?

I was not a new graduate. I was not struggling with clinical competency. I was experienced, capable, and, by most measures, successful. But I was exhausted in a way that sleep couldn't fix. I had poured myself into patients, colleagues, and a department that felt like it was running on fumes, and somewhere along the way, I had stopped feeling like a person growing and started feeling like a function that was performing.

Nobody had asked me how I was doing in a long time. Not really. Not in the way that matters.

I sat in that garage longer than I should have. And then I drove home, came back the next morning, and didn't say a word about it to anyone because there was no space for that conversation, and I wasn't sure anyone would have understood, even if there had been.

I stayed. Eventually, I found my way back to purpose, to passion, to the work that I genuinely love. But I think about that parking garage moment more than people might expect, because I know, with absolute certainty, that I am not the only one who has sat there. I know because over the years, in quiet hallways, break rooms, and parking lots of my own, I have met them. The RTs who were one bad shift away from updating their resume. The ones who had already started looking. The ones who left before anyone noticed they were struggling.

This chapter is about them. And about what we, as educators, preceptors, department leaders, could have done differently.

Meet Danielle

I'll call her Danielle.

She was two years into her career when I met her, and she was good. Not just competent. Genuinely gifted. She had the kind of clinical instincts that take some therapists a decade to develop. She connected with patients in a way that made families feel seen during the most frightening moments of their lives. Her colleagues respected her. Her patients asked for her by name.

She had also submitted her resignation letter.

I found out through the kind of informal channel that carries more truth than any official communication. A colleague mentioned it in passing, almost as an afterthought. "Did you hear Danielle's leaving?" As if it were inevitable. As if gifted people leaving was just something that happened, like the weather.

I asked if I could talk to her before her last day. She agreed, a little surprised that anyone had asked.

We sat in a small conference room with bad lighting and lukewarm coffee, and I asked her one question: What would have made you stay?

She was quiet for a moment. Then she said something I have carried with me ever since.

"I just wanted someone to notice that I was more than my assignment."

Not a raise. Not a different schedule. Not a fancy title or a bigger role. She wanted to be seen as a person with ambition, curiosity, and potential, not just as a body filling a shift. She had ideas about improving the department's weaning protocols. She wanted to pursue a specialty certification but wasn't sure the department would support it. For two years, she had felt like she was doing good work into a void, and that eventually the void had won.

Danielle left. She went to a department in another state that, within six months, had enrolled her in a leadership development program, supported her certification, and asked her to help redesign its orientation process.

She didn't need a different profession. She needed a different environment.

That distinction, between leaving the profession and leaving an environment, is the most important thing I want you to take from this chapter.

What the Data Tells Us and What It Doesn't

The workforce data on respiratory therapy retention is sobering. Depending on the source and the year, somewhere between a quarter and a third of new RTs leave the profession or change employers within their first two years. Turnover rates in allied health, particularly respiratory care, have climbed steadily in the years following the pandemic. The cost of replacing a single respiratory therapist, accounting for recruitment, onboarding, lost productivity, and the burden on remaining staff, is estimated to exceed $85,000 in many healthcare systems.

Those numbers matter. They make the business case for retention in language hospital administrators understand.

But numbers don't tell you about Danielle sitting in a conference room with lukewarm coffee. They don't capture the colleague who started calling in sick more often because she dreaded going in. They don't show you the charge therapist who was quietly applying to travel companies because he felt invisible in a department he had given six years to. The data tells us that people are leaving. It does not tell us what they needed before they did.

For that, you have to have the conversation. And in my experience, most departments do not have it, not honestly, not early enough, and not with the people who most need to be heard.

What Exit Interviews Miss

Exit interviews, when they happen at all, are one of the most well-intentioned and consistently inadequate tools in the retention conversation.

Think about the context. A person who has already decided to leave, who may be concerned about references and professional relationships, who is sitting across from someone connected to the institution they are departing from, and we ask them to tell us the truth about why they are going. Most people will give the safe answer. Schedule. Commute. An opportunity they couldn't pass up. Something that sounds neutral and forward-looking and puts no one in an uncomfortable position.

What they rarely say in an exit interview, but what they will tell you in a parking lot, or a break room, or a quiet conversation with someone they trust, is the real answer. And the real answers, collected over years of those informal conversations across multiple hospitals and states, sound less like logistics and more like this:

"I felt like I was just a number."

"Nobody ever asked me where I wanted to go."

"My preceptor made me feel stupid for not knowing things I had never been taught."

"I watched people with less experience get opportunities I never heard about."

"I was running on empty and no one noticed until I was already gone."

"I didn't feel safe speaking up. So I stopped speaking up. And then I stopped caring. And then I left."

These are not complaints about salary scales or parking. These are people telling us, with remarkable clarity, exactly what they needed and didn't receive. And if we are willing to listen, really listen, they are also telling us exactly what we need to build.

The Five Real Reasons RTs Leave

Based on workforce research and years of direct conversation with respiratory therapists at every stage of their careers, the reasons good RTs leave cluster consistently around five themes. Notice what is and is not at the top of the list.

1. No Visible Path Forward

This is the number one reason I hear, in one form or another, from RTs who are considering leaving or who have already gone. It is not that they don't love the work. It is that they cannot see where the work is taking them.

Respiratory therapy has a professional development problem that we don't talk about loudly enough. In many departments, the career path looks something like this: new graduate, staff therapist, maybe charge therapist, and then a long plateau with no clear next step unless a management position opens up. For RTs who are ambitious, curious, and growth-oriented, exactly the ones we most want to keep, that plateau feels like a ceiling.

What these RTs are not seeing is that the path forward exists. Specialty certifications, clinical ladder programs, educator roles, quality improvement leadership, preceptor development, protocol design: there is a rich professional landscape available to a respiratory therapist who knows it's there. The problem is that in too many departments, nobody has shown them the map.

Showing people the map is one of the most powerful retention tools available to us. It costs nothing except the willingness to have a conversation.

2. Feeling Unseen and Undervalued

There is a difference between being appreciated and feeling appreciated, and it matters more than most leaders realize.

An RT can receive a good performance review, be told they are doing a great job, and still feel fundamentally unseen because the recognition they received was generic, delayed, or disconnected from the specific things they had worked hardest to do. Recognition that lands is specific. It names what the person did and why it mattered. It is delivered close to the moment it was earned. And it communicates not just "good job" but "I see you, the real you, not just your output."

The RTs who feel most valued are rarely the ones in departments with the most elaborate recognition programs. They are the ones whose managers and educators know their names, remember their goals, check in on their difficult days, and occasionally say, unprompted and sincerely, "I'm really glad you're here."

That costs nothing. And its absence costs everything.

3. Poor or Absent Leadership

RTs do not leave departments. They leave leaders.

This is one of the most consistently documented findings in healthcare retention research, and it is one of the most uncomfortable truths for institutions to sit with, because it means that the solution is not a new policy or a better benefits package. It is the harder, slower work of developing leaders who actually lead.

What does poor leadership look like in a respiratory therapy department? It looks like a manager who is always available for the administrative tasks but never available for the human ones. It looks like a charge therapist who plays favorites with assignments and never addresses the tension everyone can feel. It looks like a department culture where speaking up is technically encouraged and practically punished, where the RT who raised a concern at a staff meeting finds themselves quietly sidelined in the weeks that follow.

And it looks like an educator who is so focused on competency checklists that they have lost sight of the people behind them.

Good leadership, at every level, is the single most powerful retention tool a department can develop. And leadership, like precepting, is not a quality people are born with. It is a skill that must be taught, modeled, practiced, and supported.

4. Toxic Team Culture

Culture is not what your department says it values. Culture is what your department does when things become difficult.

A department can post its mission statement on every wall and still have a culture where new RTs are talked about rather than talked to, where mistakes are punished rather than processed, where cliques determine who receives support and who gets isolated. That kind of culture is invisible from the outside and unmistakable from within.

New RTs are extraordinarily sensitive to team culture, not because they are fragile, but because they are paying attention in a way that longer-tenured staff sometimes no longer do. They notice who gets left out of conversations. They feel the chill when a certain person walks into the break room. They register, with quiet precision, whether the department's stated values match its daily behavior.

When the culture is toxic, or even just quietly unwelcoming, new RTs rarely complain loudly. They withdraw, they survive, and eventually they leave. And on their way out, they tell the safe story in the exit interview.

The antidote to toxic culture is not a team-building exercise or a new set of core values printed on a badge. It is consistent, intentional leadership behavior that models what belonging actually looks like day after day, shift after shift, in the small moments that accumulate into a culture.

5. Burnout Without a Safety Net

Respiratory therapy is one of the most emotionally and physically demanding specialties in allied health. The patient population is often critically ill. The decisions are high stakes. The pace is relentless. And the profession carries a particular kind of invisible burden: the patients who don't make it, the families who are devastated, the shifts that end with a heaviness that doesn't lift on the drive home.

Burnout in respiratory therapy is not a personal weakness. It is a predictable response to sustained high demand without adequate recovery, support, or meaning. And it accelerates dramatically when the other four factors on this list are also present, when there is no path forward, no sense of being seen, poor leadership, and a culture that does not feel safe.

What protects against burnout is not the absence of hard days. It is the presence of connection, purpose, and the sense that the hard days are shared rather than endured alone. Departments that retain their RTs through difficult stretches are departments where people feel known, supported, and part of something meaningful, even when the work is hard. Especially when the work is hard.

The Conversation Nobody Is Having Early Enough

Here is what I want to offer as a practical reframe for every educator and department leader reading this:

Retention does not begin when someone submits their resignation. It begins on day one of orientation, in the questions you ask, the investments you make, the signals you send about whether this person matters to you beyond their ability to fill a shift.

The most powerful retention conversation is not an exit interview. It is the check-in at thirty days that asks, How are you really doing? It is the conversation at six months that asks, What do you want to learn next? It is the moment at one year when you sit down with an RT and say, I see where you're going. Let me help you get there.

These conversations are not complicated. They do not require a budget approval or a committee. They require presence, intention, and the willingness to treat the people in your department as the complex, ambitious, worthy human beings that they are.

Danielle needed one of those conversations. She needed someone to ask, genuinely, what she needed and where she wanted to go. She needed to know that her ideas mattered and that her potential had been noticed. She needed a map.

She didn't get it in time. But the next Danielle in your department, and there is one, I promise you, still can.

What Staying Actually Looks Like

I want to end this chapter with something that doesn't get said enough in the retention conversation: staying is not the same as settling.

The RTs who build long, meaningful careers in respiratory therapy are not the ones who couldn't find anything better. They are the ones who found departments, educators, and leaders, who made growth possible. Who recognized their potential and named it. Who created environments where the work was hard but the support was real, where mistakes were processed rather than punished, where ambition was welcomed rather than quietly resented.

Those RTs stay not because they have no other options. They stay because they have found something worth staying for.

That is what we are building toward. Not a department that traps people through inertia, but one that earns their commitment through investment. Not retention as a metric, but belonging as a culture.

The difference between those two things is the difference between an RT who is counting down to the next opportunity and one who is growing into the best version of their professional self, right where they are, in the department you are building together.

That is the work. And it starts with understanding why people leave so we can build the kind of place they choose to stay.

Chapter Summary

- RTs rarely leave the profession. They leave environments, departments, cultures, and leadership relationships that failed to invest in them as people, not just clinicians.
- Exit interviews consistently underreport the real reasons for departure. The honest answers live in

informal conversations and require trust to surface.

- The five primary reasons good RTs leave are: no visible path forward, feeling unseen and undervalued, poor or absent leadership, toxic team culture, and burnout without a safety net. Salary is rarely the primary driver.

- Retention begins on day one of orientation, not when a resignation letter arrives. The most powerful retention tools are consistent, human, and cost nothing except intentionality.

- The goal is not a department that keeps people through inertia, but one that earns commitment through genuine investment in growth, belonging, and purpose.

Reflection Prompts

1. Think of an RT who left your department in the last two years. Based on what you know now, which of the five reasons most likely contributed to their departure? What, if anything, could have changed the outcome?

2. When was the last time you had a genuine, unhurried conversation with a staff RT, not about a patient or a task, but about how they were doing and where they wanted to go?

3. What does your department's unspoken culture communicate to a new RT in their first ninety days? How do you know?

4. Where are you on this list personally? Are you getting what you need to stay energized, growing, and connected to your purpose as an educator?

Coming Up in Chapter Four

We have spent three chapters naming the problem: the limits of orientation, the preceptor gap, and the real reasons people leave. Now we turn to the solution. In Chapter Four, we begin building the first pillar: Think. What does it actually look like to develop respiratory therapists who reason through complexity, question the plan, and bring clinical judgment to the bedside, not just clinical tasks? That is where we are going next.

"They didn't need a different profession. They needed a different environment."

04

TEACHING CLINICAL JUDGMENT IN A PROTOCOL-DRIVEN WORLD

"Knowledge tells you what to do.
Judgment tells you when, why, and for whom."

The Minimum Settings Moment

I have watched it happen more times than I can count.

It happens during competency evaluations, in simulation scenarios, and in moments designed specifically to reveal how a respiratory therapist thinks under pressure. And every time I see it, it tells me something important, not about the therapist's clinical knowledge, but about the gap between knowing a protocol and being able to reason beyond it.

Here is how it goes.

The scenario is running. The simulated patient is deteriorating, subtly at first, then unmistakably. The RT in front of me is doing everything right. They are escalating care appropriately, adjusting settings, and responding to what they see. They are thinking. You can see it happening. And then they move to the next device in the scenario, and something shifts.

They reset to minimum settings.

Not because the patient needs minimum settings. The patient in front of them is clearly telling a different story: increased work of breathing, numbers trending in the wrong direction, a clinical picture that is asking for more, not less. But the protocol says start here. And so they start here.

I watch. I let them continue. I let them verbalize their thought process out loud because, even when the reasoning is policy-driven rather than patient-driven, the act of thinking out loud is valuable, and interrupting it midstream does more harm than good. Knowing the policy matters. I don't want to take that away from them. I want to build on it.

When they finish, I don't tell them they are wrong. That is not the conversation we need to have, and frankly, it is not even accurate. They are not wrong about the protocol. The protocol is correct. What I want to explore is something more nuanced than right and wrong.

I affirm what they know first. "You know that policy well, and that matters."

And then I ask the question.

"Is that step backwards the best thing for the patient in front of you?"

I watch something happen in that pause. The shift from protocol brain to patient brain. The moment where the information they have been given, the policy, the starting point, the algorithm, meets the information in front of them, this specific patient, this specific trajectory, this specific moment in a deteriorating clinical picture, and they have to decide which one to follow.

Then I ask them to make the change they feel is best. To consider what stepping backwards might cost this patient: the possible further decompensation, the recruitment they worked so hard to achieve, the momentum of a care plan that was actually working. To weigh the policy against the person.

That conversation, that single question asked after a moment of affirmation rather than correction, is one of the most powerful clinical reasoning interventions I know. It does not make the RT feel stupid. It does not undermine their confidence in the knowledge they have worked hard to build. It simply opens a door that protocol-driven training often leaves closed:

The patient in front of you is always the primary source of information. The protocol is the starting point. Your judgment is what happens in between.

This chapter is about how we develop that judgment: deliberately, systematically, and in the real clinical environment where it actually needs to live.

Why Protocols Are Not the Problem

Before we go any further, I want to make something clear: protocols are not the enemy.

I know that, in a chapter about teaching beyond protocols, it might seem like that is where we are heading. It is not. Protocols exist for excellent reasons. They standardize care, reduce variability, protect patients from the consequences of individual inconsistency, and provide essential guidance for clinicians who are new to a setting or a patient population. A respiratory therapy department without well-designed protocols is a patient safety concern, full stop.

The problem is not the protocol. The problem is when the protocol becomes the ceiling of clinical thinking rather than the floor.

When a new RT treats a protocol as an answer rather than a starting point, when "That's what the policy says" becomes a substitute for clinical reasoning rather than a foundation for it, we have not failed to teach them the protocol. We have failed to teach them its purpose.

Protocols are built on population-level evidence. They describe what works for most patients in most circumstances. But your patient is not a population. They are a specific human being with a specific history, a specific physiology, a specific trajectory on this specific shift, and the moment that trajectory diverges from what the protocol anticipated, the RT at the bedside needs something the protocol alone cannot provide.

They need judgment.

And judgment, unlike protocol knowledge, cannot be transferred through a competency checklist or a mandatory module. It has to be developed through guided experience, structured reflection, and an educational culture that treats thinking as a clinical skill worthy of the same intentional development we give to any other skill.

The Novice-to-Expert Journey in Respiratory Therapy

Patricia Benner's foundational work on novice-to-expert development, originally written about nursing but extraordinarily applicable to respiratory therapy, gives us a useful framework for understanding why new RTs struggle with clinical judgment even when their clinical knowledge is solid.

Benner described five stages of clinical development: novice, advanced beginner, competent, proficient, and expert. What distinguishes these stages is not primarily the accumulation of knowledge. It is the development of perception. The ability to see a clinical situation not as a collection of discrete data points to be processed against a checklist, but as a whole picture with a story, a trajectory, and a meaning.

Novice clinicians see the data. Expert clinicians see the patient.

This is not a criticism of novices. It is a description of where they are in a developmental process that takes years and requires specific kinds of experience to move through. The problem in most respiratory therapy departments is not that new RTs are novices. It is that we design our orientation and education processes as if novice-to-expert development happens automatically with time and exposure, when in fact it requires deliberate, structured facilitation to accelerate.

Left entirely to their own devices, a new RT will develop clinical judgment eventually. The question is how long it takes, how many patients are cared for during that slow development, and how many of those RTs quietly disengage or leave before they ever reach the level of clinical sophistication they are capable of.

Intentional clinical reasoning education accelerates the journey. And it is not complicated, but it does require educators and preceptors who understand that their job is not just to teach RTs what to do. It is to teach them how to think.

The Three Tools That Build Clinical Reasoning

Over years of clinical education practice, I have found that the development of clinical reasoning is best supported by three specific tools, used consistently and in combination. None of them requires a simulation lab. None of them requires a budget. All of them require an educator or preceptor who is willing to be intentional about how they use the time they already have.

Tool One: Think-Aloud Precepting

Most experienced respiratory therapists have a rich, sophisticated internal monologue running during every patient encounter. They are continuously processing, integrating what they see, what they know, what they expect, and what surprises them, in a rapid, largely unconscious process that years of clinical experience have made automatic.

And they do almost all of it silently.

This is not a character flaw. It is simply what expertise looks like from the inside. The problem is what it looks like from the outside to a new RT standing beside an experienced clinician, watching them make decisions with a confidence and fluency that appears almost magical, with no visible access to the reasoning that produced it.

Think-aloud precepting is the practice of making that internal monologue external, narrating your clinical reasoning in real time so the learner beside you can hear inside a clinical mind at work.

It sounds like this:

"Before we walk in, I'm looking at these numbers and I'm noticing the respiratory rate has been trending up over the last two hours. That tells me something. I'm not sure yet if it's pain, anxiety, early respiratory compromise, or compensation for something metabolic, so when I walk in, the first thing I'm going to do is look at the patient, not the monitor. I want to see their work of breathing before I look at anything else."

Or this:

"I'm seeing a plateau pressure that's higher than I'd expect for this patient's compliance. Before I change anything, I want to rule out a few things. Is the ETT in the right position? Is there secretion buildup? Is this a patient factor or a circuit factor? Here's how I'm going to work through that..."

The new RT is not just watching a procedure. They are listening to a thought process. They are learning not only what an experienced clinician does but how they think, which is the part that competency checklists can never capture and textbooks can only approximate.

Think-aloud precepting requires practice because most experienced clinicians are not accustomed to externalizing reasoning that has become automatic. It feels awkward at first, almost performative. That discomfort is normal and temporary. The habit, once built, becomes one of the most powerful teaching tools a preceptor can carry.

Tool Two: The Predict-Assess-Debrief Cycle

Clinical reasoning is strengthened by prediction. When a learner is asked to articulate what they expect to find before they encounter a patient, they are forced to construct a mental model, to integrate everything they know about this patient's diagnosis, history, and trajectory into a coherent picture of what "should" be happening. And when reality diverges from that prediction, as it often does, the divergence becomes the most powerful learning moment of the encounter.

The Predict-Assess-Debrief cycle works like this:

Before the encounter: "Before we go in, tell me what you expect to find. Based on what you know about this patient, their diagnosis, their last set of vitals, the notes from the previous shift, what are you anticipating? What would surprise you?"

This question does something deceptively simple: it makes the learner's mental model visible. And a visible mental model can be examined, challenged, and developed in ways that an invisible one cannot.

During the encounter: Let the RT lead the assessment. Resist the urge to narrate or redirect in real time unless patient safety requires it. Let them find what they find, and notice their reaction when reality matches or diverges from their prediction.

After the encounter: "Walk me through what you expected and what you found. Where were you right? Where were you surprised? What does the difference tell you about this patient? What would you do next, and why?"

This debrief is where the reasoning develops. Not in the moment of the encounter, but in the structured reflection afterward, when the learner has space to process what happened, integrate it with what they expected, and extract the clinical lesson that lived in the gap between prediction and reality.

Done consistently, before and after every significant patient encounter, the Predict-Assess-Debrief cycle builds a habit of anticipatory thinking, one of the hallmarks of expert clinical practice. It teaches new RTs to always be asking: What does this patient's story tell me about what comes next?

Tool Three: The Reasoning Debrief: "What Could You Have Done Differently?"

Of all the clinical reasoning strategies I use, this one may be the most deceptively simple and most revealing.

It happens after the fact. After a significant clinical event, a challenging patient encounter, or a moment that didn't go the way the RT expected. I sit down with them and ask them to walk me through it. Not to evaluate them. Not to find the error. To think together.

I know that clinical reasoning has truly taken root in a new RT when two things happen simultaneously in that conversation.

The first is that they tell me their response and the outcome, not just what they did, but why they did it, what they were thinking, what they were weighing. The language shifts from task reporting ("I did this, then I did that") to reasoning narration ("I was concerned about this, so I decided to try that, because I thought it might address this"). That shift in language is a shift in thinking. You can hear it happening.

The second, and this is the one that tells me everything, is when they ask the question themselves.

"What could I have done differently?"

When a new RT arrives at that question on their own, without being prompted or corrected into it, two things have happened that no competency form can measure. They are thinking critically enough to evaluate their own performance against a standard they have internalized. And they feel safe enough in their relationship with me, and in the learning environment we have built together, to be vulnerable about their own gaps without fear of judgment.

That combination, critical thinking and psychological safety, is the soil in which clinical excellence grows. You cannot have one without the other. An RT who thinks critically but does not feel safe will keep their questions to themselves. An RT who feels safe but has not developed critical thinking will not know what questions to ask. When both are present, you have a learner who is genuinely and rapidly developing, not because you are pushing them, but because they are pulling themselves forward.

That is the moment I live for as an educator. And it does not happen by accident. It happens because someone, an educator, a preceptor, a leader, made a consistent, deliberate investment in creating the conditions where it was possible.

Building Psychological Safety: The Invisible Infrastructure

I want to spend a moment on psychological safety because it is the foundation on which all three of these tools rest, and without it, none of them work.

Psychological safety, as defined by researcher Amy Edmondson, is the belief that one will not be punished or humiliated for speaking up with ideas, questions, concerns, or mistakes. In a clinical education context, it means the new RT believes, based on consistent evidence from the people around them, that not knowing something is an invitation to learn rather than an occasion for judgment.

This sounds simple. It is not easy to build, and it is remarkably easy to destroy.

A single moment of dismissiveness from a preceptor, an eye roll, an impatient sigh, a response that makes the new RT feel stupid for asking, can undo weeks of careful relationship building. A culture where mistakes are processed publicly rather than privately, where questions are treated as interruptions rather than opportunities, where the unspoken message is you should already know this, that culture produces RTs who go silent when they are uncertain. And silent uncertainty at a bedside is a patient safety concern.

Building psychological safety is not about removing all difficulty or discomfort from the learning environment. Some discomfort is productive: the stretch of being asked to reason through something hard, the productive struggle of working at the edge of your current capability. What psychological safety removes is the fear. The fear of being judged, embarrassed, or dismissed. That fear is the enemy of clinical reasoning development because it is the enemy of honest questioning, and honest questioning is how reasoning grows.

As an educator, you build psychological safety through consistency. Through being the person who always responds to a question with genuine engagement rather than impatience. Through handling mistakes in private, with curiosity rather than criticism. Through asking "what were you thinking?" before you offer what you would have done. Through celebrating the RT who says "I wasn't sure, so I asked" at least as enthusiastically as you celebrate the RT who got it right.

And through the small, cumulative acts of human decency that communicate, shift after shift: This is a safe place to not know things yet. We are building something here, together, and your growth matters to me.

A Note on the Protocol and the Person

I want to return, one final time, to the new RT who reset to minimum settings during the competency scenario.

After our conversation, after the question, after the pause, after the moment where protocol brain met patient brain, something shifted. Not dramatically. Not all at once. But visibly.

They looked at the simulated patient in front of them. They considered what that patient was telling them. And they made a different decision, not because I told them the policy was wrong, but because I asked them to weigh the policy against the person. To hold both pieces of information at the same time and decide which one, in this moment, for this patient, should lead.

That is clinical judgment. Not the absence of protocol knowledge. The integration of it. The ability to know the rule and know when the situation calls for something more than the rule can provide.

That ability is not innate. It is developed. It is developed by educators and preceptors who ask the right questions, who create the conditions where reasoning can grow, and who understand that the most important thing they can teach a new RT is not what to do when everything goes according to plan.

It is how to think when it doesn't.

Chapter Summary

- Protocols are the floor of clinical practice, not the ceiling. The goal of clinical reasoning education is to help new RTs integrate protocol knowledge with patient-specific judgment, not to replace one with the other.
- Novice-to-expert development in respiratory therapy is not automatic. It requires deliberate facilitation: specific tools, structured reflection, and an educational culture that treats thinking as a clinical skill.
- Think-aloud precepting makes the invisible visible by narrating clinical reasoning out loud so learners can hear inside an expert mind at work.
- The Predict-Assess-Debrief cycle builds anticipatory thinking by asking learners to construct and examine mental models before and after every significant patient encounter.
- The Reasoning Debrief, anchored by the question "What could you have done differently?", reveals clinical reasoning development and psychological safety simultaneously. When a new RT asks that question on their own, both things are present.
- Psychological safety is the invisible infrastructure that makes all clinical reasoning development possible. It is built through consistency, curiosity, and the daily communication that this is a safe place to not know things yet.

Reflection Prompts

1. Think about the last time you watched a new RT follow a protocol when the patient in front of them was telling a different story. How did you respond? Looking back, what question could you have asked that would have opened the door to clinical reasoning rather than simply correcting the decision?

2. How often do preceptors in your department think aloud during patient encounters? What would it take to make that a consistent practice?

3. When was the last time a new RT came to you and asked what they could have done differently without being prompted? What does your answer tell you about the psychological safety in your learning environment?

4. Where in your current orientation or education process is clinical reasoning development explicitly addressed, not just clinical skill performance? If it isn't, where could you begin to build it in?

The Three Clinical Reasoning Tools
Quick Reference: Reproducible for preceptor training or Preceptor Power Hour use

Think-Aloud Precepting. Before or during a patient encounter, narrate your reasoning out loud. Starter phrase: "Before we walk in, here's what I'm thinking and why..."

Predict-Assess-Debrief. Before: "What do you expect to find, and what would surprise you?" During: Let the RT lead. Observe without redirecting unless safety requires it. After: "Walk me through what you expected, what you found, and what the difference tells you."

The Reasoning Debrief. After a significant encounter or event: "Tell me what happened, what you were thinking, what you decided, and what you might do differently." Wait for them to ask the last question themselves. When they do, celebrate it.

Coming Up in Chapter Five

We have built the foundation of clinical reasoning development and the tools that make it possible. In Chapter Five, we go deeper into the think-aloud approach, exploring how preceptors can develop the specific language and habits that make reasoning visible, and how educators can coach preceptors to become more intentional teachers of clinical thought.

"The patient in front of you is always the primary source of information. The protocol is the starting point. Your judgment is what happens in between."

05

THE THINK-ALOUD REVOLUTION

"To teach is to learn twice." – *Joseph Joubert*

Before You Walk In

She was a new graduate in a general care area, one of those foundational rotations that experienced clinicians sometimes underestimate precisely because it isn't the ICU, isn't the NICU, isn't the high-stakes environment where the drama is visible and the stakes are obvious.

But here is what general care teaches, when it is taught well: normal. And knowing normal, truly, deeply, clinically knowing what a well-perfused, comfortably breathing, appropriately oxygenating patient looks and sounds and feels like, is the foundation on which every other clinical judgment is built. You cannot recognize abnormal quickly and accurately if you have never learned to see normal clearly. The ICU will come. The ventilator will come. The 3 am deterioration will come. But if the foundation is not solid, none of what comes later will stand on it the way it needs to.

Her preceptor understood this. And on this particular morning, before they walked into their first patient room together, the preceptor stopped.

"Before we go in," she said, "tell me what you think we're going to find."

The new graduate paused. And then she answered in the only language she had available to her at that stage of her development, the language of tasks.

"I'm going to put on the pulse oximetry probe. Listen to breath sounds. Put the medication in the nebulizer cup."

She was not wrong. Those things needed to happen. But the preceptor heard something important in that answer, not incompetence, but a window into how this new RT was organizing her clinical world. She was thinking in actions, not in assessments. In tasks, not in pictures. She knew what to do. She did not yet know what to see.

The preceptor made a decision in that moment that changed the entire shape of the orientation that followed.

Instead of walking into the room and demonstrating the tasks, which would have been easier, faster, and entirely consistent with how most preceptors operate, she stayed in the hallway for a few more minutes and did something different.

She talked.

She narrated what she expected to find when they walked through that door. She described what a patient on this medication, with this diagnosis, at this point in their treatment should look like: the anticipated work of breathing, the expected breath sounds, the color and affect and posture that would tell her, before she touched a single piece of equipment, whether this patient was doing what she expected or something else entirely.

And then they walked in together, and the new graduate, for the first time, entered a patient room with a picture already forming in her mind rather than a checklist forming in her hands.

That is the think-aloud revolution. Not a technique. Not a protocol. A fundamental shift in how preceptors understand their role: from demonstrators of clinical skill to narrators of clinical thought.

The Automation Problem

Here is the honest truth about why think-aloud precepting does not happen naturally in most respiratory therapy departments:

Experience makes it hard.

This sounds counterintuitive. We tend to assume that the most experienced clinicians make the best teachers precisely because of their experience. And in many ways, they do. But experience does something to clinical reasoning that creates a specific and significant teaching challenge: it makes reasoning automatic.

The respiratory therapist who has assessed thousands of patients does not consciously work through each step of a pulmonary assessment the way a new graduate does. They walk into a room and they know, with a speed and a wholeness that feels almost intuitive, what they are looking at and what it means. The integration of observation, history, pathophysiology, and clinical pattern recognition that once required deliberate, step-by-step effort has, through years of repetition, become a single fluid act.

This is the hallmark of expertise. It is also, from a teaching perspective, a problem.

Because when reasoning becomes automatic, it becomes invisible. The expert clinician is no longer aware of the steps they are taking; they have been compressed into something that feels like instinct. And invisible reasoning cannot be transferred. A new RT standing beside an expert who is operating on clinical autopilot sees the output of the thinking, the decision, the action, the adjustment, but has no access to the process that produced it. They see the magic trick without seeing the mechanics. And no matter how many times they watch the trick, they cannot reproduce it until someone shows them how it works.

Donald Schön, in his landmark work *The Reflective Practitioner*, described this phenomenon as the gap between knowing-in-action and reflection-in-action: the difference between the tacit knowledge that drives expert performance and the conscious, articulable knowledge that can be shared and taught. Bridging that gap, making tacit knowledge explicit, is precisely what think-aloud precepting is designed to do.

The other reason think-aloud precepting does not happen naturally is simpler and more fundamental: nobody ever told preceptors it was their job.

This is not a criticism. It is an observation about a systemic gap. Most preceptors were assigned their role because they were good clinicians, and then left to figure out the teaching part on their own. The model they were given, explicitly or implicitly, was: demonstrate the skill, have the orientee repeat it, evaluate whether they did it correctly.

That model produces task competency. It does not produce clinical reasoning. And most preceptors have never been offered an alternative, not because they wouldn't use one, but because nobody sat them down and said: here is what teaching clinical thinking actually looks like, and here is how you do it.

That conversation is what this chapter is designed to start.

Think-Aloud Develops Two People at Once

Here is something that surprises preceptors the first time they hear it, and that experienced educators already know:

Think-aloud precepting develops the preceptor as much as it develops the orientee.

This is not a side effect. It is one of the most important features of the practice. And understanding it changes the way preceptors approach the think-aloud work, from something they do for the orientee to something they do with the orientee, for both of them.

Here is why.

When you ask a preceptor to narrate their clinical reasoning out loud, you are not just asking them to share what they think. You are asking them to examine what they think, to slow down the automatic process, pull it apart, and reconstruct it in language that someone else can follow. That act of reconstruction is itself a form of reflection. And reflection, as Schön argued, is one of the most powerful mechanisms for professional growth available to any practitioner at any stage of their career.

But there is something even more revealing at work here, and I want to say it directly, because it is one of the most important insights in this book:

The same respiratory therapists who revert to policy minimum settings when a patient in front of them needs more are also preceptors.

Read that again.

The task-driven thinking we identified in Chapter Four, the tendency to follow the protocol rather than read the patient, does not disappear when someone becomes a preceptor. It does not automatically resolve with years of experience. An RT who has never been challenged to articulate the reasoning behind their clinical decisions can spend an entire career making those decisions competently without ever examining why they make them. And when that RT is assigned an orientee and asked to teach, they teach what they know how to do: tasks, because that is the language they have always used to describe clinical practice.

When you ask that preceptor to think aloud, something important happens. They have to find words for reasoning that may have always been wordless. And in finding those words, or discovering that the words are not there, that "Because that's what the protocol says" is the best explanation they can produce, they encounter their own clinical reasoning in a new way.

Sometimes that encounter is illuminating. The preceptor discovers that their reasoning is richer and more sophisticated than they realized, that the automatic process, when slowed down and examined, reveals a depth of clinical pattern recognition that they never had occasion to articulate before. That discovery is energizing. It changes how they see themselves as clinicians and as teachers.

And sometimes the encounter is challenging. The preceptor discovers gaps in their own reasoning, places where they have been following the map without looking out the window, places where the protocol has been standing in for clinical judgment without either of them noticing. That discovery is uncomfortable. And it is one of the most valuable things that can happen to a preceptor, because a preceptor who examines their own reasoning is a preceptor who keeps growing. And a preceptor who keeps growing is a preceptor whose orientees thrive.

Being able to explain the why is not just a teaching skill. It is a clinical skill. And the think-aloud practice develops both simultaneously.

What Think-Aloud Actually Sounds Like

One of the barriers to think-aloud precepting is that preceptors are not sure what it is supposed to sound like. They imagine it as a formal narration, clinical and precise, like a textbook brought to life, and the gap between that imagined standard and their actual thought process feels too large to bridge.

The reality is both simpler and more powerful than that. Think-aloud precepting sounds like a clinician thinking out loud. It is allowed to be imperfect, exploratory, and honest. In fact, the imperfection is part of what makes it valuable, because a new RT who hears an experienced clinician say "I'm not sure yet, here's how I'm going to figure it out" learns something that no textbook can teach: that uncertainty is a normal part of clinical practice, and that what separates experienced clinicians from inexperienced ones is not the absence of uncertainty but the ability to navigate it systematically.

Here are examples of what think-aloud precepting sounds like in practice, not as scripts to be memorized, but as illustrations of the kind of narration that makes reasoning visible:

Before entering a general care patient room:

"Before we go in, I'm building a picture of this patient in my head. She's 68, with COPD exacerbation, has been on 2 liters by nasal cannula since yesterday. Based on that, I'm expecting to find someone who is breathing a little harder than normal, maybe some accessory muscle use, and possibly pursed-lip breathing. I want to hear whether her breath sounds are clear or if there's wheezing, because that will tell me whether we're dealing with bronchospasm on top of the exacerbation or if it's more of an air-trapping picture. And I'm going to look at her face before I look at her monitor, because her face will tell me how hard she's working before the numbers do. What are you expecting to find?"

During a ventilator assessment in the ICU:

"I'm looking at this waveform, and something is catching my attention. See how the flow curve isn't returning to baseline before the next breath? That tells me there's air trapping happening. Now I need to figure out why. Is it the rate? The I:E ratio? Is this patient's intrinsic PEEP building up? Before I change anything, I want to do a quick expiratory hold and see what we're actually dealing with. Here's what I'm thinking as I do that..."

After an unexpected finding:

"Okay, that was not what I expected. I was anticipating clear breath sounds on the right after the repositioning, but I'm still hearing diminished breath sounds. That tells me either the repositioning wasn't enough or there's something else going on that I need to think about. Let me walk you through what I'm considering and why..."

When uncertain:

"I want to be honest with you: I'm not completely sure what I'm seeing here yet. Here's what I know, here's what I don't know, and here's how I'm going to work through it. Watch what I do and tell me if you see something I'm missing."

That last example is especially important. A preceptor who models uncertainty navigated systematically, rather than certainty performed, gives their orientee permission to be uncertain too. And an orientee who feels permission to be uncertain will ask questions. And an orientee who asks questions develops faster than one who performs with a confidence they do not yet have.

Teaching Preceptors to Think Aloud

Knowing that think-aloud precepting is valuable and knowing how to do it are two different things, and most preceptors need guided practice before the habit feels natural.

Here is a progression I use with preceptors in Preceptor Power Hours and individual coaching conversations:

Step One: Awareness. Start by asking the preceptor to reflect on their own clinical reasoning process. "When you walk into a patient room, what are you actually thinking about before you touch anything? Walk me through it." Most preceptors have never been asked this question. The process of answering it, of pulling their automatic reasoning into conscious language, is itself the first step toward being able to share it.

Step Two: Low-Stakes Practice. Ask the preceptor to think aloud with a colleague before trying it with an orientee. Role-play a patient scenario and have them narrate what they are thinking as they work through it. This removes the pressure of the real clinical environment and gives them space to find their words without an audience that depends on them.

Step Three: The Pre-Encounter Narration. Start with just the hallway conversation, the two minutes before entering the room. Ask preceptors to build the habit of stopping before every patient encounter and sharing with their orientee what they expect to find and why. This is the lowest-stakes version of think-aloud and the easiest entry point. It requires no disruption to the clinical workflow and produces immediate results.

Step Four: In-the-Moment Narration. Once the pre-encounter narration feels natural, expand to narrating during the encounter: at decision points, during unexpected findings, when something requires an adjustment. Not a running commentary of every action, but a voiced thought at the moments where reasoning is happening.

Step Five: Debrief and Reflect. After the encounter, ask the preceptor: "What did you find yourself thinking that you didn't say out loud? What was hardest to put into words?" This reflection deepens the preceptor's own clinical self-awareness and identifies the places where their reasoning is most automatic, which are also the places their orientee most needs to hear it.

The Foundational Assessment Argument

I want to return for a moment to the new graduate in the general care area, because the setting of her story matters as much as the story itself.

General care is where foundational assessment skills live. And foundational assessment skills are, in my experience, one of the most underinvested areas of respiratory therapy education, precisely because they don't seem as dramatic as what happens in the ICU.

But here is what I have learned over twenty years of clinical practice across every RT setting: you cannot recognize abnormal quickly if you have never learned to see normal deeply. The RT who has spent genuine time in general care, who has assessed hundreds of patients who are breathing adequately, oxygenating appropriately, and moving air without significant effort, has built an internal reference library that the RT who fast-tracked to critical care simply does not have.

When something goes wrong at 3 am in the ICU, the RT who knows normal in their bones will catch it faster. Not because they are smarter. Because they have a baseline so deeply internalized that deviation registers immediately, in the face, in the work of breathing, in the quality of the breath sounds before the monitor has time to alarm.

Think-aloud precepting in the general care setting is not a consolation prize for not being in the ICU. It is the construction of the foundation on which everything else is built. And a preceptor who understands that, who can communicate to a new graduate that "we are here to learn what normal is, because that knowledge will follow you into every critical care environment you ever work in," is giving that new RT something that will serve them for the rest of their career.

When You Know It's Working

The moment I know think-aloud precepting has truly taken hold in a preceptor is not when the orientee improves.

It is when the preceptor tells me it made them a better clinician.

That testimony, and I have heard versions of it more times than I can count, is the most powerful evidence I know that think-aloud precepting is doing something deeper than teaching. It is the preceptor telling me that the act of making their reasoning visible changed how they see their own practice. That slowing down to explain the why revealed aspects of their clinical thinking that years of automatic practice had obscured. That teaching their orientee to see the patient rather than the protocol made them look at the patient more carefully too.

This is the multiplier effect of think-aloud precepting. One educator, working with one preceptor, who begins to narrate their reasoning with one orientee, and suddenly two clinicians are forming where only one was intended. The preceptor did not come to the Preceptor Power Hour expecting to discover gaps in their own clinical reasoning. They came to learn how to teach. And what they found was that teaching and learning, done this way, are not separate activities. They are the same activity, experienced from different sides of the same conversation.

Joseph Joubert wrote that to teach is to learn twice. In think-aloud precepting, that is not a metaphor. It is a mechanism. And it is one of the most quietly revolutionary things happening in the departments that have embraced it.

Chapter Summary

- Think-aloud precepting is the practice of narrating clinical reasoning out loud during patient encounters so that learners can access the thinking behind the action, rather than just the action itself.
- Experience makes think-aloud precepting difficult because expertise compresses reasoning into

automaticity. Making automatic reasoning explicit requires deliberate practice and is a learnable skill.

- Most preceptors do not think aloud naturally for two reasons: their reasoning has become too automatic to narrate without effort, and nobody ever told them that teaching reasoning was part of their job.
- Think-aloud precepting develops the preceptor as much as the orientee. When experienced clinicians are asked to explain the why behind their decisions, they examine their own reasoning and sometimes discover that the reasoning is richer; at other times, they find it shallower. Both discoveries produce growth.
- The same task-driven thinking that causes new RTs to follow protocols mechanically exists in preceptors too. Think-aloud precepting interrupts that pattern in both simultaneously.
- Foundational assessment in general care settings is not a lesser clinical experience. It is the construction of the normal-recognition baseline that makes rapid abnormal detection possible in every critical care environment that follows.
- You know think-aloud precepting is working when a preceptor tells you it made them a better clinician, not just a better teacher.

Reflection Prompts

1. Think about your own clinical reasoning process. When you walk into a patient room, what are you actually thinking before you touch anything? Have you ever put that into words for yourself or for someone else?

2. Which of the barriers to think-aloud precepting, automaticity or lack of role clarity, is most prevalent among your preceptors? What would address it most directly?

3. When was the last time a preceptor in your department told you that teaching made them a better clinician? If that conversation hasn't happened, what might it take to create the conditions where it could?

4. How is foundational assessment in general care settings valued and communicated in your department? Do new RTs understand why it matters, not just what they are doing, but what they are building?

Think-Aloud Starter Phrases

A Preceptor Reference Card

Reproducible for preceptor training or Preceptor Power Hour use

Before the encounter: "Before we go in, here's what I'm expecting to find and why..." "Based on what I know about this patient, I'm thinking..." "What would surprise me walking into this room is..."

During the encounter: "I'm noticing _____ and it's making me think about _____..." "Before I change anything, I want to rule out..." "This isn't what I expected. Here's how I'm working through it..."

When uncertain: "I'm not sure yet. Here's how I'm going to figure it out..." "I want to think this through out loud. Tell me if you see something I'm missing."

After the encounter: "What did you expect to find? What surprised you?" "Walk me through what you were thinking while we were in there." "What question is still sitting with you after that encounter?"

Coming Up in Chapter Six

We have built the think-aloud practice and explored why it simultaneously develops both the preceptor and the orientee. In Chapter Six, we introduce the Clinical Reasoning Passport. This ninety-day tool makes learning visible over time, turning the daily practice of clinical reflection into a documented developmental journey that both the new RT and the educator can examine, celebrate, and build upon together.

"To teach is to learn twice, and in
think-aloud precepting,
that is not a metaphor. It is a mechanism."

06

THE CLINICAL REASONING PASSPORT

Making Growth Visible, One Entry at a Time

"We do not learn from experience.
We learn from reflecting on experience."
– John Dewey

The Day She Looked Back

It was a routine check-in, the kind that happens at the sixty-day mark of orientation, when the initial intensity has settled and the new RT has found enough footing to start asking bigger questions about where they are and where they are going.

She came prepared, which, in itself, was already different.

She walked in with her passport open, not waiting for me to ask about it, not treating it as a form to be handed over and reviewed, but holding it the way you hold something that belongs to you. Something you have been thinking about. She had a specific entry she wanted to talk about, a case from week three that she had written about when it happened and then returned to at the thirty-day milestone with fresh eyes.

She pointed to her early entry. The language was task-focused, a list of what she had done, in order, with brief notes about whether each step had gone correctly. Standard new graduate documentation. Competent. Careful. And almost entirely without reasoning.

Then she pointed to what she had written about the same case four weeks later.

It was a different document entirely. Not because the facts had changed. The patient, the intervention, and the outcome were all the same. But because she was a different clinician looking at them. The second entry asked questions the first entry hadn't known to ask. It connected the patient's presentation to the pathophysiology in ways that four more weeks of clinical experience had made possible. It identified, with a clarity that surprised even her, two moments in that early case where she had done the right thing for the wrong reason, where the outcome had been correct but the reasoning had been incomplete.

She looked up at me and said something I have not forgotten:

"I didn't realize how much I didn't know when I thought I was doing fine."

That sentence is the Clinical Reasoning Passport in a single line. Not a criticism of where she was in week three; she was exactly where a new graduate should be. But a revelation of how much invisible growth had happened between week three and week seven, growth that no competency checklist had captured and no supervisor observation had surfaced, because it was happening inside, in the quality of her thinking, in the depth of her clinical questions, in the gradual construction of a reasoning framework that was becoming, week by week, more sophisticated and more her own.

The passport made that growth visible. And seeing it changed how she understood herself as a clinician.

But the passport does something else too, something less celebratory and more essential. It catches what is hidden. And sometimes what is hidden is not growth. It is a gap.

What the Passport Reveals That Nothing Else Does

Competency checklists tell you what a new RT can do. Supervisor observations tell you what they do when someone is watching. Preceptor feedback tells you how they perform on the floor in real time.

None of these tools tell you what a new RT thinks when they are alone with a patient and nobody is observing. None of them reveal the internal reasoning, or the absence of it, that drives the decisions being made at the bedside every shift.

The Clinical Reasoning Passport does.

Because the passport asks new RTs to write, and writing, unlike task performance, cannot be faked. A new RT who is genuinely reasoning through a clinical situation will produce documentation that reflects that reasoning, that shows the integration of observation, pathophysiology, decision-making, and reflection that characterizes developing clinical judgment. And a new RT whose thinking is still primarily task-focused, even when their task performance looks competent, will produce documentation that reveals that gap in ways that no checklist ever could.

I discovered this not in theory, but in practice, when I reviewed a passport entry from a new RT who had been receiving positive feedback from their preceptor. On the floor, they appeared confident. Their tasks were completed correctly and on time. Their preceptor had no significant concerns.

The passport entry told a different story.

The new RT had documented a patient encounter in detail: the steps they had taken, the interventions they had performed, the outcome that had followed. But when I read the entry looking for reasoning rather than action, something was missing. There was no why. No consideration of alternatives. No acknowledgment of what the patient's presentation had told them before they intervened, or what it told them after. The documentation was a record of events, not a record of thought.

That gap, invisible on the floor, invisible in the preceptor relationship, invisible in every formal assessment tool the department had, was visible in the passport. And seeing it early, at week four rather than week fourteen, meant we could address it while there was still time and space to build what was missing.

That is what the passport is for. Not surveillance. Not evaluation. Discovery of growth and of gaps, in time to do something about both.

What the Clinical Reasoning Passport Is

The Clinical Reasoning Passport is a structured, portable document that a new RT carries through their first ninety days. It is not a journal in the casual sense; it has specific prompts and a specific structure designed to surface clinical reasoning rather than simply record clinical events. And it is not a competency form; it is not signed off, it is not pass/fail, and it is not something that is done to the new RT. It is something they do with their own developing clinical mind, guided by an educator who reviews it regularly and uses it as the foundation for meaningful developmental conversation.

The passport has three components that work together to capture the full picture of a developing clinician:

Component One: Weekly Case Reflections

Once a week, or after any significant patient encounter that warrants deeper examination, the new RT documents a case using a structured reflection framework. Not a narrative summary of what happened, but a guided analysis that asks:

What did I observe when I first encountered this patient? What did those observations tell me?

What did I decide to do, and why? What alternatives did I consider?

What happened? Did the outcome match my expectations? If not, why not?

What would I do differently if I encountered this patient again tomorrow?

What question is this case leaving me with that I haven't yet been able to answer?

That last question, what question is this case leaving me with, is one of the most diagnostically useful prompts in the entire passport. A new RT who consistently produces rich, specific unanswered questions is a new RT whose clinical curiosity is alive and growing. A new RT who consistently writes "none" or produces vague, generic responses is a new RT whose reflection practice needs more support and whose clinical reasoning may be more superficial than their floor performance suggests.

The weekly case reflection is the engine of the passport. It is where the most visible development happens and where the most important gaps are revealed.

Component Two: The Question Log

This component addresses something that every educator who has worked with new RTs knows well: the questions they don't ask out loud.

New RTs have more questions than they voice. They have questions they are afraid will make them look incompetent. Questions they started to ask and then stopped when they sensed impatience. Questions that surfaced at 2 am during a solo shift, when no one was available to ask. Questions they didn't even know they had until a patient did something unexpected and they realized, in a moment of quiet uncertainty, that they didn't know why.

The Question Log is a running record of those questions, a private space where the new RT can write down what they are genuinely uncertain about without fear of judgment. It is reviewed by the educator, not as a measure of deficiency but as a map of the learner's growing awareness of their own knowledge boundaries.

This matters for two reasons.

First, it surfaces learning needs that formal assessment never captures: specific clinical concepts, equipment questions, pharmacology gaps, and pathophysiology uncertainties directly relevant to the patients this RT is caring for right now. The Question Log transforms those hidden needs into a targeted, personalized education agenda.

Second, it normalizes uncertainty as a professional condition. When a new RT writes their questions down and sees them on paper, reviewed by an educator who responds with engagement rather than judgment, they learn that not knowing is not a failure. It is the starting point of every clinical question that has ever moved the profession forward.

That lesson, internalized early, produces the kind of clinician who asks questions throughout their whole career rather than performing confidence they don't always have.

Component Three: Goal Tracking, 30, 60, and 90 Days

On day one of orientation, before the clinical work begins, the new RT sits down with the passport and sets three goals. Not performance goals, not "pass the vent competency" or "complete arterial line training." Development goals. Goals that reflect who they want to become as a clinician, not just what they want to be able to do.

"I want to be able to walk into a patient room and know, before I touch anything, what I expect to find and why."

"I want to feel confident asking a physician to reconsider a plan when I think the patient needs something different."

"I want to understand ventilator graphics well enough to explain what I'm seeing to a family member."

These goals are revisited at thirty days, sixty days, and ninety days, not to evaluate whether they have been achieved, but to examine how the new RT's relationship with their own goals has evolved. Sometimes a goal that seemed important on day one has been surpassed by day thirty and needs to be replaced with something bigger. Sometimes a goal that seemed straightforward reveals itself to be more complex and more meaningful than the new RT initially understood. Sometimes a goal surfaces a need that the formal orientation plan had not anticipated.

The goal-tracking component does something that no externally imposed competency timeline can do: it puts the new RT at the center of their own development. It communicates, from the very first day, that their growth is not something being done to them by the institution. It is something they are doing, with guidance, with support, and with a document in their hands that belongs to them and tells the story of who they are becoming.

How It Works in Practice

The passport is introduced on day one, not as a form to be completed but as a tool to be used. The framing matters enormously. A new RT who receives the passport with the message "this is how we track your development" will treat it as documentation. A new RT who receives it with the message "this is how you will see your own growth" will treat it as theirs.

Brief weekly entries happen throughout the ninety days: case reflections after significant encounters, question log updates whenever uncertainty surfaces, brief notes about goals as they evolve. These do not need to be long. A well-constructed case reflection of two or three paragraphs is more valuable than a page of narrative summary. The prompts are specific enough to guide brevity toward depth.

At the thirty-day milestone, the educator sits down with the new RT and the passport together. Not to evaluate. To explore. "What are you noticing about your own thinking? What cases are staying with you? What questions are surfacing that you weren't expecting?" This conversation is qualitatively different from a standard orientation check-in because the passport gives it substance. There is something on the table, something the new RT has produced, something that reflects their inner clinical life in a way that a performance review never could.

The sixty-day review, like the one that opened this chapter, is often where the most powerful growth revelations happen, when the new RT has enough distance from their early entries to see them clearly and enough development to understand what they were missing.

The ninety-day close is both a celebration and a transition. The passport doesn't end at ninety days because development ends. It ends because the new RT has established the reflective habit that the passport was designed to build. The goal is not a document they complete and hand in. It is a practice they carry forward: asking why, examining their own thinking, and treating every patient encounter as an opportunity to learn something that will serve the next patient better.

When New RTs Meet the Passport

I want to tell you about the response I most commonly see when new RTs receive the passport for the first time, because it reveals something important about what is missing in most orientation experiences.

They are surprised that someone is asking.

Not surprised by the tool itself. By the question behind it. The question that the passport represents: What are you thinking? What are you uncertain about? What do you want to become?

Most new RTs arrive at their first job having been asked, repeatedly and in many forms, what they can do. Can you set up a ventilator circuit? Can you perform a bronchodilator treatment? Can you pass the competency? Those are the questions the system has taught them to expect and to answer with performance rather than reflection.

Nobody has asked them what they are thinking. Nobody has given them a space for their questions that don't feel like a test. Nobody has invited them, in a structured and supported way, to set their own development goals and be held to them with curiosity rather than judgment.

When the passport does those things, when it communicates through its very structure that the new RT's inner clinical life matters, that their uncertainty is welcome, that their goals are theirs, something shifts. They do not treat it as extra work. They treat it as an invitation.

And then something even more remarkable happens. They bring it to check-ins. They walk in with it open, with entries flagged, with questions they want to discuss. The passport stops being something the educator reviews and becomes something the new RT drives. The conversation shifts from "let me tell you how you're doing" to "here is what I've been thinking, what do you see that I'm missing?"

That shift, from passive recipient of feedback to active driver of their own development, is the moment the passport has done its deepest work. It is the moment a new RT stops being someone orientation is happening to and becomes someone who is genuinely, intentionally, irreversibly growing.

A Note on Resistance, and What It Tells You

Not every new RT immediately embraces the passport. Some find the reflective writing uncomfortable, not because they are not thinking, but because they have never been asked to examine their thinking before, and the process feels unfamiliar and exposed.

This resistance is information.

A new RT who struggles to write a case reflection, who produces task summaries when asked for reasoning analysis, who writes "I felt confident" when asked what they were thinking at the moment of a clinical decision, is showing you something important about how they have been taught to understand their own practice. Not a character flaw. Not a deficiency. A gap in reflective development that the passport is specifically designed to address.

The response to this resistance is not to lower the bar, to accept task summaries, and move on. It is to sit with the new RT and model the reflection process. To take one of their entries and work through it together. "You wrote that you administered the treatment as ordered. Tell me, what was the patient doing before you walked in that made you think the treatment was necessary right now? What did you expect to hear when you listened to their breath sounds afterward? Were you right?"

Those questions, asked with genuine curiosity, in a psychologically safe space, begin to build the reflective vocabulary that the passport requires. And a new RT who starts with task summaries and ends the ninety days with genuine clinical analysis has not just improved their documentation; they have also developed a fundamentally different relationship with their own practice, one that will serve them and their patients for the rest of their career.

Chapter Summary

- The Clinical Reasoning Passport is a structured, portable ninety-day document that makes a new RT's clinical thinking visible, revealing both growth and gaps in ways that competency checklists and supervisor observations cannot.
- The passport has three components: weekly case reflections guided by specific reasoning prompts, a running question log for uncertainties that don't get voiced out loud, and goal tracking revisited at thirty, sixty, and ninety days.
- Brief weekly entries are combined with deeper milestone reviews, creating a rhythm of reflection that builds the habit of examining one's own practice rather than simply performing it.
- New RTs typically embrace the passport because nobody has ever asked them to reflect before. When they begin bringing it to check-ins and driving the conversation themselves, the passport has done its deepest work.

- Resistance to the passport is information, a signal that reflective practice needs modeling and support, not that the bar should be lowered.
- The goal of the passport is not a document that gets completed and handed in. It is a reflective habit that gets carried forward into every patient encounter, every clinical decision, and every stage of a developing RT's career.

Reflection Prompts

1. What does your current orientation process do to make a new RT's clinical thinking visible, not just their clinical performance? Where are the gaps?
2. Think about a new RT who appeared to be doing well on the floor but surprised you later with a reasoning gap you hadn't anticipated. What might a passport have revealed earlier?
3. When was the last time you asked a new RT what they were uncertain about in a space where they felt genuinely safe enough to answer honestly? What did they tell you?
4. What would it take to introduce a version of the Clinical Reasoning Passport in your department? What would you need to adapt it to your specific context and population?

The Clinical Reasoning Passport Template
Reproducible. Adapt freely for your department's context and population.

NEW RESPIRATORY THERAPIST: CLINICAL REASONING PASSPORT

90-Day Developmental Record

Name: ____________________

Start Date: ______________

Educator: ____________________

DAY ONE – My Starting Point

Three development goals for my first 90 days. Not task goals, growth goals.

Goal 1:

____

Goal 2:

____

Goal 3:

____

One thing I am most uncertain about as I begin:

One thing I am most excited to learn:

WEEKLY CASE REFLECTION

(Complete after any significant patient encounter. Brief is fine; depth matters more than length.)

Date: ____________

Patient situation (no identifying information):

____

What did I observe that told me this patient needed attention?

What did I decide to do, and why? What alternatives did I consider?

What happened? Did it match what I expected?

What would I do differently next time?

What question is this case leaving me with?

MY QUESTION LOG
(Running record of uncertainties, clinical, procedural, relational. Nothing is too small.)

Date | My Question | How I Found the Answer (or who helped me)

30-DAY MILESTONE REFLECTION

Looking back at my Day One goals, where am I with each one?

What has surprised me most in my first 30 days?

What am I still most uncertain about?

What do I need more of in the next 30 days?

60-DAY MILESTONE REFLECTION

Read your earliest case reflections. What do you notice about how your thinking has changed?

What clinical concept has become clearer, and what made it click?

Where do I still feel like I'm following the map instead of reading the patient?

Updated or new goal for the final 30 days:

90-DAY MILESTONE REFLECTION

What kind of clinician am I becoming? Describe yourself, not your skills, but your thinking.

What is the most important thing you learned in these 90 days that no textbook taught you?

What question are you carrying into the next stage of your career?

What do you want your preceptor or educator to know about what this experience meant to you?

"We do not learn from experience.
We learn from reflecting on experience.
The passport is where that reflection lives."

6B

LEVEL UP: BECAUSE DEVELOPMENT DOESN'T STOP AT ORIENTATION

"You don't build a culture of learning for new hires inside a department where everyone else stopped being asked to grow."

It Hit Different

He pulled me aside after it was over.

He was an experienced respiratory therapist, the kind of clinician who has seen enough, done enough, and survived enough to have earned a healthy skepticism about department initiatives. He had walked into Level Up Week with the particular energy of someone who has attended many competency events and expects this one to be exactly like the others: a checklist, a signature line, and an hour of his life he will not get back.

What he found was something else entirely.

He told me he enjoyed it. That it challenged him to think a little deeper. That he had learned updates to policies he thought he already knew, not because the policies had been handed to him on a form, but because he had been asked to work through them at a station, out loud, with colleagues beside him asking the same questions he was. He mentioned the team building. He mentioned the energy in the room. And then he said something that I wrote down afterward because I knew it mattered:

"It was refreshing. It hit different. I hope we do something like this more than once a year."

That sentence told me everything I needed to know about what Level Up Week had accomplished, and about the gap it had revealed.

Not a gap in clinical knowledge. A gap in clinical engagement. A gap between what experienced respiratory therapists are capable of when they are genuinely challenged and what most annual competency processes ask of them. A gap that most departments have stopped noticing because they stopped expecting anything different.

This chapter is about closing that gap. Not just for new hires. For everyone.

The Staff Development Problem Nobody Talks About

We spend a great deal of time in respiratory therapy education, in this book and in the field generally, talking about developing new RTs. Orientation. Preceptor relationships. Clinical reasoning tools. Ninety-day plans. All of it important. All of it necessary.

And then there is everyone else.

The staff respiratory therapist who has been in the department for four years. The charge therapist with a decade of experience. The Tier Four preceptor who knows this department better than almost anyone. The RT who was exceptional once and has quietly plateaued. The one who is still exceptional and has no idea how much further they could go.

What does your department's development system offer them?

In most departments, the honest answer is: annual competency. A checklist. Skills station with a supervisor holding a clipboard. Perhaps a mandatory module or two. The same process, year after year, that measures whether staff can still perform the skills they were verified on during orientation, without ever asking whether their thinking has grown, whether their practice has evolved, or whether they have anything left to learn that the department has not yet offered them.

This is not a criticism of competency verification. As we established in Chapter One, competency is the floor. It matters. It must happen.

But the floor is not the ceiling. And for experienced staff, clinicians who cleared the competency floor years ago and have been standing on it ever since without anyone offering them a ladder, the annual competency process communicates something damaging without intending to:

We only need you to stay the same.

Level Up Week communicates something entirely different. And the fact that experienced staff respond to it the way they do, with energy, with engagement, with voluntary attendance, tells us that the hunger for meaningful development never disappears. It just stops being fed.

What Level Up Week Is

Level Up Week is an annual, simulation-based competency preparation event that replaces the traditional competency checklist model with a station-based, reasoning-focused experience that challenges every staff member, new graduate, and twenty-year veteran alike, to think deeply, ask questions, and engage with clinical content in a way that a signature line never could.

Here is how it works.

Staff arrive at the simulation lab with a passport. This physical document travels with them through the event, station by station, capturing their questions, their reflections, and their engagement at each stop. The passport is not a test; it is a record of thinking. It communicates, from the moment staff pick it up, that what happens today is not about checking boxes. It is about learning.

The stations are hosted not just by the clinical educator but by supervisors, charge therapists, and Tier Four preceptors, the most experienced and most trusted clinicians in the department. This decision is intentional and important. When a Tier Four preceptor hosts an NIV station and walks their colleagues through not just the equipment setup but the clinical reasoning behind device selection and parameter adjustment, two things happen simultaneously: the attendees learn from someone they respect, and the host deepens their own mastery through the act of teaching. The think-aloud revolution described in Chapter Five plays out at a department-wide scale.

The stations themselves cover the clinical content that staff engage with every day, but from a reasoning-first perspective rather than a task-first one:

NIV Station. Not just mask fit and circuit setup, but: When do you choose NIV over high flow? What does your patient need to tell you before you initiate? What does failure look like, and how early can you recognize it?

High Flow Nasal Cannula Station. Not just flow rates and FiO_2, but: What is the physiological mechanism? When is high flow the bridge, and when is it the destination? What are you watching for that tells you it's working?

Ventilator Graphics Station. Not just waveform identification, but: What is this graphic telling you about this patient's lungs right now? What would you change and why? What does this pattern mean for your next decision?

Equipment Setup Station. Not just assembly, but: What could go wrong? How would you know? What does a malfunctioning circuit look like from the patient's perspective before it looks wrong on the monitor?

Pulmonary Vasodilator Station. Not just protocol, but: What is the pathophysiology driving this therapy? What are you hoping to see? What tells you it's working, and what tells you it isn't?

At every station, policies are present, not hidden, not forbidden, but available as a reference rather than a crutch. The goal is not to remove policy knowledge from the conversation. It is to ensure that policy knowledge is integrated with clinical reasoning rather than substituted for it. Staff are expected to know the policy, explain why it exists, and describe when the patient in front of them might require something more than the policy alone can provide.

That expectation, applied to experienced staff as much as to new graduates, is what makes Level Up Week different from every competency event that came before it.

It Wasn't Mandatory. They Still Came.

I want to pause here and say something plainly.

Level Up Week was not mandatory.

Let that settle for a moment. In a profession where mandatory attendance is sometimes the only reliable mechanism for getting staff into a training room, Level Up Week drew strong attendance without requiring it. Experienced therapists showed up. Tier Four preceptors showed up and hosted stations. New graduates came not knowing what to expect and left energized. The survey feedback was outstanding, not the polite, neutral feedback of people completing a required form, but the specific, enthusiastic feedback of people who felt genuinely seen and genuinely challenged.

Voluntary attendance at a well-designed development event is one of the most powerful signals a department culture can produce. It says: *People here want to grow. When we offer something worth showing up for, they show up. The culture of development we are building is taking root.*

Carol Dweck's research on growth mindset, the belief that abilities can be developed through dedication and hard work, tells us that environments shape mindset as much as individual disposition does. A department that consistently offers meaningful development opportunities does not just serve the staff members who already have a growth mindset. It cultivates that mindset in staff who have been living in a fixed-mindset environment for years, staff who have stopped expecting to be challenged and, when challenged, discover that the desire to grow was never gone. It was just waiting for an invitation.

Level Up Week is that invitation.

New Graduates and Veterans: One Room, One Culture

One of the things that struck me most about the first Level Up Week was watching new graduates and experienced staff move through the stations together.

New graduates arrived with uncertainty, not knowing what to expect or how they would measure up to colleagues with years of more experience. Experienced staff arrived with skepticism, not sure this would be worth their time or whether there was anything left to learn they hadn't already seen.

What happened in the room surprised both groups.

The new graduates discovered that experienced colleagues had questions too, that not knowing everything is not a new graduate problem but a clinical reality that never fully resolves, no matter how many years you have been practicing. That discovery did something important for their confidence. It normalized uncertainty as a professional condition rather than a personal deficiency.

And the experienced staff discovered that the new graduates, the ones they might have dismissed as inexperienced, as not yet knowing enough to contribute, were asking questions that pushed the discussion in directions nobody had anticipated. The fresh eyes of a new graduate, unencumbered by the habits and assumptions that accumulate with years of practice, sometimes see things that experience has learned to overlook.

That cross-generational, cross-experience-level energy in the room was not accidental. It was the product of a design that deliberately brought everyone together rather than separating development by seniority. And it produced something that no tier-specific training could have generated: a shared experience. A common reference point. A moment that the whole department could point to and say, "We did that together."

That is culture building. And it happened at a competency event.

The Ecosystem: Level Up Week and Preceptor Power Hours Together

Here is what I want you to see about Level Up Week that goes beyond the event itself.

It does not stand alone.

Level Up Week feeds directly into the Preceptor Power Hour that follows it. Staff who have just spent time reasoning out loud at stations, who have just been asked to verbalize their why in front of colleagues, arrive at the next Preceptor Power Hour already primed for the think-aloud conversation. They have experienced what it feels like to be asked to explain their reasoning rather than just demonstrate their skill. They understand, from the inside, what that experience produces in the learner. And they are ready, in a way that a purely theoretical discussion could never produce, to take that practice back to their orientees.

This is the ecosystem at work.

Level Up Week develops the whole department. Preceptor Power Hours develop the preceptors specifically. The Clinical Reasoning Passport develops the individual new RT over ninety days. And the think-aloud practice connects all three, because it is the common language of the culture being built. A culture where reasoning is visible, where questions are welcomed, where explaining the why is expected of everyone at every level of experience.

When these elements work together, which they do, by design, the result is not just a better orientation program. It is a different kind of department. One where development is not something that happens to new hires and then stops. Where it is woven into the fabric of how the team operates, how competency is approached, how preceptors are prepared, and how staff understand their own professional identity.

That kind of department does not just develop better RTs. It keeps them.

Building Your Own Level Up Week: Where to Start

I want to be practical here because I know that reading about a well-executed event is very different from imagining how to build one in your own department with your own constraints.

Here is what you need, and what you do not need.

You need: A simulation space or any room that can accommodate stations. It does not need to be a formal sim lab. A conference room with equipment pulled from the department works. Clinical content organized around reasoning questions rather than task checklists. A passport document, simple, one or two pages, that travels with each staff member. Station hosts who are respected by their peers: supervisors, charge therapists, experienced preceptors. A survey at the end. And the willingness to let go of the checklist as the primary evidence of learning.

You do not need: A large budget. Mandatory attendance policy. Administrative approval for a multi-week planning process. Perfect execution on the first attempt.

Start with two or three stations. Run it for half a day. Survey your staff afterward and let their feedback shape the next iteration. The experienced therapist who pulled me aside after our first Level Up Week did not experience a flawlessly executed, perfectly designed event. He experienced something that respected his expertise, challenged his thinking, and made him feel like his development still mattered.

That is achievable in any department. With any budget. Starting with the staff and the equipment you already have.

The passport, the stations, the reasoning questions, these are tools. The real thing you are building is a message. And the message is this:

Development does not stop when orientation ends. It does not stop at five years. It does not stop at ten. You are still growing. And this department is invested in that growth, not just for the new hire in bay four, but for every single person on this team.

When your staff believe that message, when they feel it, when they see it in the events you design and the questions you ask and the voluntary attendance at something worth showing up for, you will have built something that no retention strategy, no compensation package, and no HR initiative can replicate.

You will have built a place people choose to stay.

Chapter Summary

- Staff development does not end at orientation, and a department that invests only in new hire development communicates to experienced staff that their growth no longer matters. That message is a retention risk.
- Level Up Week is an annual, simulation-based competency-preparation event that replaces task-checklist verification with station-based, reasoning-focused learning for the entire department, not just new hires.
- Stations are hosted by supervisors, charge therapists, and Tier Four preceptors, making the event a peer learning experience as much as an educator-led one.
- Voluntary attendance speaks louder than any survey result. When staff come because they want to, because the event respects what they know and challenges them to go deeper, it signals that a culture of development is taking root.
- Level Up Week feeds directly into Preceptor Power Hours: staff who have reasoned out loud at stations arrive at the next Power Hour already primed for the think-aloud conversation.
- The ecosystem of Level Up Week, Preceptor Power Hours, and the Clinical Reasoning Passport creates a department-wide culture of reasoning, reflection, and growth, not just a better orientation program.

- You do not need a large budget or a perfect plan to begin. You need two or three stations, a passport document, respected station hosts, and the willingness to ask your staff to think rather than just demonstrate.

Reflection Prompts

1. What does your department currently offer experienced staff in terms of meaningful development, beyond annual competency verification? How do you think they would describe it if asked honestly?
2. Think about your most experienced RT. When was the last time something in their professional environment genuinely challenged them to think more deeply? What was it, and what did it produce?
3. If you ran a Level Up Week in your department tomorrow with what you currently have, what would the stations be? Who would host them?
4. Where are the natural connection points between your existing education activities? How could they feed each other more intentionally, the way Level Up Week feeds into Preceptor Power Hours?

Level Up Week Planning Guide: Quick Reference
Reproducible for department education planning

Before the Event:

- Identify 3–6 clinical stations based on current competency requirements and department learning needs
- Select station hosts from supervisors, charge therapists, and experienced preceptors
- Design reasoning-first questions for each station, not "can you do this?" but "why would you do this, and when?"
- Create the passport document: simple, portable, one page per station
- Communicate the purpose clearly: this is not a test. It is a learning experience.

During the Event:

- Have policies available at every station, as reference, not as answers
- Require verbalization: staff must explain their reasoning, not just demonstrate their skill
- Encourage peer discussion between staff at each station
- Capture energy and questions in real time; these will shape next year's event

After the Event:

- Survey every attendee with specific questions about what challenged them, what they learned, what they want more of
- Share results with the department; transparency about feedback builds trust
- Use survey themes to inform the next Preceptor Power Hour topic
- Begin planning next year's event while the energy is still in the room

Coming Up in Chapter Seven

We have built the clinical reasoning tools for individual learners and the development ecosystem for the whole department. In Chapter Seven, we turn to the LEAD pillar, beginning with the foundational argument that leadership in respiratory therapy is not a title, not a promotion, and not something that happens to a select few. It is a capacity that lives in every RT in your department right now, and your job is to find it, name it, and grow it.

"Development does not stop when orientation ends. And a department that stops investing in its people, at every level, has already started losing them."

07

LEADERSHIP IS NOT A TITLE

"The most dangerous leadership myth is that leaders are born, that there is a genetic factor to leadership. That's nonsense; in fact, the opposite is true. Leaders are made rather than born."
– Warren Bennis

NOW HIRING: Bedside RT Leader
No Application Required. You Already Have the Job.

POSITION TITLE: *Bedside Respiratory Therapy Leader*
DEPARTMENT: *Wherever You Are Right Now*
SHIFT: *All of them. But especially the hard ones.*
REPORTS TO: *The patient in front of you. Also the family who hasn't slept in four days. Also the nurse who just called you for the third time this hour. Also your own conscience at 3 am.*
SALARY: *The same as before. Sorry about that.*

POSITION SUMMARY:

We are seeking a dynamic, committed professional to serve in a critical leadership role within our respiratory care department. This position requires no formal title, no office, no business cards, and no parking spot with your name on it. What it does require is showing up, fully, consistently, and with the kind of presence that makes the people around you better.

PRIMARY RESPONSIBILITIES:

- *Advocate clearly and confidently for patients when the plan isn't working, even when the person you're advocating to has more letters after their name than you do*
- *Mentor the new graduate on your shift who is quietly terrified and will not admit it, not because it's your job description, but because you remember what that felt like*
- *Speak up in rounds when you have information the team needs, even when you weren't technically asked*
- *Make a clinical decision under pressure at 2 am with no supervisor available and own it completely*
- *Teach a patient's family how to use a nebulizer with the patience of someone who has never explained it before, even though you have explained it four hundred times*
- *Model professionalism in the break room when the conversation turns toxic, which it will*
- *Challenge a protocol that isn't serving your patient, document your reasoning, and escalate appropriately, because that is what an advocate does*
- *Show up for your colleagues on the hard days in ways that have nothing to do with your assignment*

- *Know when you don't know something, say so out loud, and find the answer instead of guessing*
- *Leave every patient room having done not just the right thing, but the right thing for this patient, right now, for reasons you could explain to anyone who asked*

QUALIFICATIONS:

- *Active RRT or RRT-eligible (preferred but not required; students, we see you too)*
- *Genuine investment in patient outcomes*
- *The ability to hold clinical confidence and personal humility at the same time*
- *A working understanding that being right matters less than being helpful*
- *Some tolerance for ambiguity, because medicine has a great deal of it*

EXPERIENCE REQUIRED: *Whatever you have. It is enough to start.*

BENEFITS:

- *The satisfaction of knowing you changed something today that the chart will never fully capture*
- *Occasional unsolicited gratitude from patients and families that will stay with you longer than any performance review*
- *The respect of colleagues who notice, even when they don't say so*

- *A professional identity that belongs to you, not to whoever signs your paycheck*

TO APPLY:

You already have. Every shift you showed up for. Every patient you advocated for. Every colleague you helped without being asked. Every moment you chose to do the harder right thing instead of the easier wrong one.

Congratulations. You're hired.

Now, can we talk about why you don't believe it yet?

The Management Myth

Ask most respiratory therapists, especially new ones, what leadership means, and you will hear some version of the same answer.

A manager. A supervisor. A director. Someone with a title on a door and a schedule that doesn't involve nights and weekends. Someone who goes to meetings instead of running codes. Someone who, frankly, sounds more like a different job than a different level of the same one.

This is the management myth. And it is one of the most limiting beliefs in the respiratory therapy profession, not because management is bad, but because equating leadership with management means that every RT who does not want to be a manager has unconsciously decided that leadership is not for them. That the influence, the advocacy, the mentorship, the clinical courage that defines genuine professional leadership, all of it, belongs to someone else. Someone with a title. Someone further up the org chart. Someone who is, by implication, more important.

The management myth does not just limit individual RTs. It limits departments. When leadership is understood as a positional attribute rather than a behavioral one, departments end up with a small number of people carrying the entire weight of professional culture, the managers and supervisors who are officially responsible for leading. Meanwhile, a vast reservoir of untapped leadership capacity sits on the floor every shift, unrecognized and undeveloped, wearing scrubs and a stethoscope.

That is an enormous waste. And it is entirely unnecessary.

Because leadership, real leadership, the kind that changes patient outcomes and shapes department culture and makes new RTs feel like they belong somewhere worth staying, does not live in the office. It lives at the bedside. It lives in the choices made at 2 am when nobody is watching. It lives in the colleague who stays fifteen minutes after their shift to help a new graduate understand something that wasn't clicking. It lives in the RT who speaks up in rounds even when their voice shakes.

It lives in your department right now. In people who have no idea that what they are doing has a name.

Your job, as an educator and a leader, is to give it one.

What Leadership Actually Looks Like in Respiratory Therapy

Let me be specific, because abstract definitions of leadership have a way of staying abstract. Here is what leadership looks like in the lived reality of a respiratory therapy department:

It looks like the RT who speaks up. Not loudly. Not confrontationally. But clearly, with clinical evidence, at the moment when something important needs to be said. The RT who flags a deteriorating patient before the monitor alarms. Who questions a ventilator order that doesn't match what they see at the bedside. Who advocates in rounds for a patient who cannot advocate for themselves. That is leadership. It requires clinical knowledge, professional courage, and the judgment to know when and how to use both.

It looks like the RT who teaches without being asked. The one who notices a new graduate struggling with a concept and takes five minutes, not because it's their assignment, not because anyone is watching, to sit down and explain it. The one who shares a clinical pearl at shift change because they think it will help. The one who debriefs a difficult case with a colleague because they know that processing matters. Teaching is one of the most powerful forms of leadership available to any clinician at any level. It requires neither title nor authority. It requires only the willingness to invest in someone else's growth.

It looks like the RT who models culture. Every department has informal culture carriers, the people whose behavior sets the tone for what is acceptable, what is expected, and what kind of place this is to work. These are not always the managers. They are often the staff RT with eight years of experience whose attitude in the break room influences ten other people. The one who treats every patient like they matter, every family like they're terrified, every new colleague like they belong. Culture is not built in policy documents. It is built in the daily choices of the people who show up, and the informal leaders who model what those choices should look like.

It looks like the RT who stays curious. The one who asks why after they already know what. Who reads the latest AARC clinical practice guideline not because a competency requires it but because they want to know. Who brings a question from their own practice to a Preceptor Power Hour because they are genuinely trying to get better. Curiosity is a form of leadership because it raises the standard, not just for the individual but for the culture around them. A team that includes curious, growth-oriented clinicians becomes more curious and growth-oriented.

It looks like the RT who shows up for people. Not just for patients. For colleagues. The one who notices that a teammate is having a hard shift and checks in. Who remembers that the new graduate has their first solo weekend coming up and sends an encouraging text. Who advocates in a staff meeting for a scheduling change that would benefit the night shift, even though they work days. This is not soft leadership. This is the kind of human investment that builds the psychological safety and belonging that makes departments worth staying in.

None of these behaviors require a title. All of them require a choice. And all of them are available to every respiratory therapist in your department, right now, regardless of where they are on the career ladder.

The RT Leadership Ladder Revisited

In the introduction to this book's LEAD section, I described a five-level RT Leadership Ladder, a framework for understanding how leadership develops across a clinical career, from the earliest professional voice of a new graduate to the formal leadership of a supervisor or director.

I want to revisit it here with more depth, because the ladder is not just a descriptive framework. It is a developmental tool. And understanding where each RT in your department sits on it is the first step toward helping them climb.

Level One: Professional Voice. This is where every RT begins. Level One leadership is the practice of speaking up, documenting thoughtfully, advocating clearly, and engaging professionally. It does not require experience. It requires the decision to show up as a professional rather than just as a shift worker. Many new RTs arrive at this level naturally, and some experienced RTs, for reasons worth exploring, have never fully claimed it.

Level Two: Active Mentorship. Level Two is where the RT begins investing deliberately in someone else's development. The preceptor. The peer coach. The experienced RT who takes a new graduate under their wing informally, outside the official preceptor relationship, because they remember what it felt like to need someone who wasn't busy. Level Two leadership multiplies impact because the investment made here ripples forward through every person the mentee goes on to influence.

Level Three: Informal Influence. Level Three RTs are the go-to people. The ones colleagues turn to when they are not sure what to do. The charge RT. The resource therapist. The person whose opinion matters in the room, even when the supervisor is present. Level Three influence is earned, not assigned, and it is some of the most powerful leadership in any department because it operates through trust rather than authority.

Level Four: Program Champion. Level Four is where clinical leadership becomes structural. The RT who leads a protocol revision. Who chairs a quality improvement initiative. Who serves as a Tier Four preceptor and takes genuine ownership of the department's development culture. Level Four leaders are the bridge between the clinical floor and the formal leadership team, and they are among the most valuable people in any department.

Level Five: Formal Leadership. Supervisor. Manager. Director. The title on the door. This is where the management myth places all leadership, and where, in reality, only a fraction of it lives. Level Five matters. But it is built on the four levels beneath it. A Level Five leader who skipped Levels Two, Three, and Four will struggle in ways that no management training can fully address.

The question for every educator reading this is not: how do I develop more Level Five leaders? It is: how do I help every RT in my department claim the level they are ready for, and grow toward the next one?

Naming It Out Loud

Here is something I want to ask you to do, and I am asking you to do it this week, not someday.

Find an RT in your department who is leading without knowing it. The one who teaches without being asked. Who speaks up when it matters. Who shows up for colleagues in ways that nobody officially tracks. Who is, by every meaningful measure, a leader, and who would look at you with genuine surprise if you called them one.

And call them one.

Not in a performance review. Not in an annual competency. In a hallway, or a break room, or a quiet moment after a shift. Specifically, with evidence. "I noticed what you did today when you stayed to help Marcus figure out that waveform. That's what leadership looks like. I want you to know I see it."

Watch what happens.

In my experience, one of two things occurs. Either the RT is genuinely surprised because nobody has ever used that word about them before, and hearing it opens something, or they are quietly not surprised at all because, somewhere beneath the humility, they already knew and having it named out loud gives them permission to own it.

Either response is the beginning of something. A shift in identity. A new way of understanding what they are already doing. A reason to keep doing it, more intentionally, more visibly, more confidently.

This is how leadership cultures are built. Not through training programs alone, not through competency requirements, not through org chart restructuring. Through the accumulation of moments in which someone in authority looks at someone who doesn't think they qualify and says, clearly and specifically: I see you leading. Keep going.

You have that authority. Use it this week.

A Note to the RT Who Is Reading This and Thinking "Not Me"

I know you are out there.

You are reading this chapter and nodding along when it describes other people, the colleague who speaks up in rounds, the RT who mentors without being asked, the go-to person everyone trusts. You are nodding because you recognize them. And you are simultaneously, quietly, not applying any of it to yourself.

I want to say something directly to you.

Go back and read the job posting at the beginning of this chapter. Read every responsibility on that list. And ask yourself, honestly, without the self-protective instinct to minimize, how many of those things you have done in the last thirty days.

Not perfectly. Not always. But genuinely, in the way that counts.

If the answer is most of them, and I suspect it is, then you are already leading. The only thing missing is your permission to call it that.

Leadership is not something that happens to you when you get a title. It is something you choose, shift by shift, in the small decisions that add up to the kind of clinician and colleague you are becoming.

You are already becoming it.

Own it.

Chapter Summary

- The management myth, the belief that leadership equals management, is one of the most limiting ideas in respiratory therapy. It causes RTs who don't want to be managers to opt out of leadership entirely, leaving vast reserves of clinical and cultural influence untapped.
- Leadership in respiratory therapy lives at the bedside. It looks like speaking up, teaching without being asked, modeling culture, staying curious, and showing up for people, none of which require a title.
- The RT Leadership Ladder provides a five-level framework for understanding and developing leadership across a clinical career, from Professional Voice to Formal Leadership. Every RT is on the ladder. Your job is to help them climb.
- Naming leadership out loud, specifically, with evidence, in the moment, is one of the most powerful developmental interventions available to

any educator. It shifts identity. It gives permission. It builds the culture.

- Leadership is a choice made shift by shift. Every RT in your department is already making it. The question is whether they know it.

Reflection Prompts

1. Think about the three most influential people in your department. How many of them have formal leadership titles? What does your answer tell you about where leadership actually lives?
2. Who in your department is leading without a title right now, and have you told them? What is stopping you from having that conversation this week?
3. Where do your staff RTs sit on the Leadership Ladder? Pick three people and place them honestly. What would it take to help each one move to the next level?
4. When you think about your own leadership journey, how long did you lead before someone gave it a name? What did it mean when they finally did?

Coming Up in Chapter Eight

We have established that leadership lives at every level of the department, and that the most important thing an educator can do is find it, name it, and grow it. In Chapter Eight, we turn to the most critical and most underdeveloped leadership relationship in respiratory therapy: the preceptor. Because before we can grow leaders across the department, we need to develop the people who are already leading the most vulnerable members of it, one orientation at a time.

"Leadership is not something that happens to you when you get a title. It is something you choose, shift by shift, in the small decisions that add up to the kind of clinician you are becoming."

08

PRECEPTOR POWER HOURS

The Chapter That Didn't Exist Anywhere Else, Until Now

"You can't teach what you don't know.
But you also can't teach what you've never been shown how to share."

The Chin Check

I want to tell you about the moment I knew Preceptor Power Hours were working.

It didn't happen during a session. It happened in a hallway, in the middle of an ordinary workday, when one of my preceptors pulled me aside to have a conversation about a situation she was navigating with her orientee.

She was describing how she had approached a feedback conversation, one that had been difficult, one where she had been tempted to either soften the message so much it lost its meaning or deliver it so directly it landed like a verdict. And as she talked, I realized she was narrating back to me, almost word for word, a framework we had discussed together in a Preceptor Power Hour session weeks earlier. She had internalized it. She had applied it. And now she was holding me accountable to the same standard in our conversation.

She gave me, as she would later laughingly describe it, a chin check.

I loved every second of it. Because that is exactly what transformation looks like. Not a preceptor who attended a session and filed the handout away. A preceptor who took a tool, made it her own, and was now using it so naturally that she could turn it back around on the person who taught it to her, with confidence, with warmth, and with just enough humor to keep the whole thing from getting too serious.

That hallway moment is why this chapter exists. And it is why, if you take nothing else from this book, I hope you take this: developing preceptors is not optional. It is the lever that moves everything else.

The Missing Link

We have discussed in previous chapters the gap between clinical and teaching excellence, how being a great respiratory therapist does not automatically make someone a great preceptor, and how assigning the teaching role without preparing people for it is one of the most consequential mistakes a department can make.

But knowing the problem exists and knowing what to do about it are two different things. And for a long time, the honest answer to "what do we do about it?" was: not much. A brief orientation to the preceptor role, perhaps. A form to fill out. An expectation that experience would fill in the gaps.

Preceptor Power Hours are my answer to that gap. They are not a curriculum. They are not a certification program. They are not another mandatory module to click through. They are something simpler and, I would argue, more powerful than any of those things: a dedicated, recurring space where preceptors can come together to learn, to reflect, to struggle honestly, and to grow, as teachers, as leaders, and as people.

There is nothing quite like them in the respiratory therapy literature, which is exactly why I am writing this chapter.

Building the Foundation: A Tiered Preceptor System

Before Preceptor Power Hours can do their best work, the right architecture needs to be in place. And in my department, that architecture is built on a principle that sounds simple but changes everything: not every preceptor is right for every orientee, and pretending otherwise sets both of them up to struggle.

This is why I developed a tiered preceptor system. It is the structural backbone that makes everything else, the Power Hours, the feedback loops, the intentional development, possible.

Here is how it works.

Tier One preceptors work primarily with students in general care areas. They tend to be earlier in their own careers, experienced enough to teach foundational skills, but close enough to the student experience to remember what it felt like to not know things yet. That proximity matters more than most people realize. A student who is overwhelmed in their first clinical rotation does not need the most seasoned therapist in the department. They need someone who can meet them where they are, speak their language, and make the learning environment feel safe rather than intimidating.

Tier Two preceptors work with extern students, students on critical care rotations, and new graduates entering the residency program. These preceptors have deeper clinical experience and a stronger command of complex patient populations. They are comfortable in the ICU, comfortable with ambiguity, and comfortable guiding a learner through the kind of high-stakes encounters that define early RT practice.

Tier Three preceptors work specifically with experienced new hires: RTs who are coming in with existing clinical knowledge and need a different kind of orientation. Not "here is how to be an RT" but "here is how we do things here, here is our culture, here is what we expect, and here is how your experience fits into what we are building." The skill set required for this tier is different, less about teaching clinical fundamentals and more about integration, culture orientation, and peer-level professional relationship building.

Tier Four preceptors are the most versatile and the most developed. They can work with any new hire at any level and are typically assigned as mentors rather than simply preceptors. They are the preceptors who have demonstrated not just clinical excellence but genuine teaching excellence, the ones whose orientees consistently thrive, who model the Developer approach described in Chapter Two, and who, through the Preceptor Power Hour process, have grown into something approaching master educators.

Preceptors choose their tier; they are not assigned to it. That choice matters because ownership changes everything. A preceptor who has selected the population they want to work with is far more invested in doing that work well than one who has been assigned to a role without input.

But choice is not the only factor. Supervisors and I review and approve tier placements because self-assessment, while important, is not always accurate. A preceptor who wants to move into Tier Four because of the status it carries, but who has not yet developed the teaching skills that tier requires, is not doing their orientees any favors. The approval process exists to ensure that tier placement reflects genuine capability, not just aspiration, and to create a growth path that makes Tier Four something worth working toward.

The Assignment Behind the Assignment

There is a layer of intentionality in how I make preceptor assignments that does not appear on any form or policy document, and it may be one of the most important things I do.

I match personalities.

Not perfectly; that would require a level of omniscience I do not possess and a scheduling flexibility that hospital staffing does not permit, but intentionally, thoughtfully, and with the specific goal of creating conditions where learning is most likely to happen.

Some orientees need a preceptor who is calm and methodical, someone whose steady presence helps regulate the anxiety of a new clinical environment. Others need energy and enthusiasm, someone who makes the work feel exciting rather than overwhelming. Some need directness. Some need warmth first. Some need a preceptor who has walked a similar path, who came from the same kind of program, who navigated similar challenges, who can say "I remember feeling exactly like that" and mean it.

I also make assignments with burnout prevention in mind. Precepting is demanding work, and a preceptor who has just come off an intensive orientation with a struggling orientee needs time to recover before taking on the next assignment. Rotating preceptors thoughtfully, giving people space between assignments, matching workload to capacity, and paying attention to signs of fatigue is not just being kind. It is strategically essential. A burned-out preceptor is not a good preceptor, no matter how skilled they are. And losing a great preceptor to burnout is a loss the department feels for a long time.

Two-Way Feedback: The Daily Pulse

One of the most powerful and most underused tools in preceptor development is feedback that flows in both directions, not just from preceptor to orientee, but from orientee to preceptor as well.

In my department, we use daily evaluations. Every day during orientation, the orientee evaluates the preceptor and the preceptor evaluates the orientee. Both evaluations are reviewed by me.

This structure does several things simultaneously.

It gives me real-time information. I do not have to wait until a mid-orientation check-in to discover that a preceptor relationship is struggling, that an orientee is feeling unsupported, or that a particular dynamic is developing that needs to be addressed. I can see it in the daily feedback: a pattern of ratings that shifts, a comment that signals friction, a discrepancy between what the preceptor is reporting and what the orientee is experiencing, and I can intervene while there is still time to course-correct.

It gives preceptors data about their own teaching. Most preceptors receive almost no feedback about how they are doing as teachers. The daily evaluation changes that. When a preceptor consistently sees that their orientee feels unclear on the reasoning behind clinical decisions, or conversely, that their orientee consistently rates their explanations as the most valuable part of the shift, that information shapes how they show up the next day in ways that no amount of classroom instruction can replicate.

It gives orientees a voice. New RTs are in a position of significant vulnerability during orientation, dependent on their preceptor for learning, for evaluation, and often for their sense of whether they are going to make it. Giving them a daily mechanism to provide feedback about their own experience, anonymized enough to feel safe, visible enough to matter, communicates that their perspective is valued and that their orientation is a two-way relationship, not something being done to them.

And it normalizes feedback as a daily practice rather than a formal event. When evaluation is something that happens every day, briefly, simply, as a matter of course, it loses the weight and the anxiety that tend to accumulate around less frequent, higher-stakes assessments. Both the preceptor and the orientee get comfortable with the rhythm of honest reflection, which is exactly the culture we are trying to build.

What a Preceptor Power Hour Is, and What It Isn't

Let me be specific, because I have found that when people hear "preceptor development session," they immediately picture one of two things: a formal training with slides and learning objectives, or an informal venting session that ends with everyone feeling validated but nothing actually changing.

Preceptor Power Hours are neither of those things, although they contain elements of both, held in careful balance.

What they are:

A Preceptor Power Hour is a monthly, sixty-minute structured session designed specifically for active preceptors. Not for all staff. Not for new RTs. For the people whose job it currently is to guide, teach, and develop someone else, and who are doing that job on top of their regular patient assignment, often without anyone asking how it's going.

The session is facilitated by the clinical educator, that's you, and its purpose is threefold: to equip preceptors with practical tools they can use immediately, to create a space where the real challenges of precepting can be named and addressed honestly, and to build a sense of community among the people doing this work so that they feel connected rather than isolated.

What they are not:

They are not a complaint forum, although honest conversation about difficulty is welcome and necessary. They are not a performance review, although growth and accountability are woven throughout. They are not optional in spirit, even when they are not mandatory on paper. And they are absolutely not something that can be replaced by an email or a handout, because the relational and communal elements are inseparable from the learning.

The Architecture of a Session

One of the questions I get most often when I describe Preceptor Power Hours is: What actually happens during the hour?

The honest answer is: it depends. Some sessions are planned in advance around a specific topic. Others emerge from what is happening in the department right now: a challenging orientation, a pattern the educator has noticed, a question that keeps surfacing in one-on-one conversations. The best sessions are often a mix of both: a planned framework that provides structure, and enough flexibility to follow the conversation where it genuinely needs to go.

Here is the general architecture I have found works well:

Welcome and Check-In (5–10 minutes). Start by taking the room temperature. Asking simple questions like, *"How is your current orientation going? What's one word that describes where you are right now?"* does two things simultaneously. It gives you real-time information about what your preceptors are carrying, and it signals to them that this is a space where how they are doing matters, not just what they are doing.

This is not a small thing. Most preceptors go through their entire precepting experience without anyone asking how it's going for them. Starting every session with that question consistently and intentionally communicates that the person doing the teaching is as important as the person being taught.

Topic and Discussion (35–40 minutes). This is the heart of the session. The topic might be planned, feedback skills, clinical reasoning instruction, managing the struggling orientee, or it might be responsive to something the check-in surfaced. Either way, the goal is not to lecture. It is to facilitate.

Ask more than you tell. Present a scenario and ask how preceptors would handle it before offering any framework. Use real situations, anonymized, handled with care, as discussion anchors. Let preceptors teach each other, because peer learning in this context is extraordinarily powerful. The preceptor who has navigated a difficult orientee relationship and come out the other side has wisdom that no educator's slide deck can replicate.

Tool or Takeaway (10 minutes). Every session should end with something concrete, a framework, a phrase, a one-page resource, a specific approach that the preceptor can take back to the floor and use immediately. This is non-negotiable. People are busy. They have given you an hour. Send them back with something tangible that makes that hour feel worthwhile.

Close and Preview (5 minutes). End by naming what was accomplished, not in a performative way, but genuinely. "What I heard today was..." Then preview the next session topic so preceptors leave already thinking about it.

The Badge, and Why It Matters More Than You Think

I want to tell you about a specific badge moment that I will never forget.

She was a Tier Four preceptor now. But for a long time, she insisted that precepting was not her ministry. Her words, delivered with the particular conviction of someone who has made peace with a decision and is not interested in revisiting it.

And she was not wrong, exactly. When she was assigned to precept outside of her preferred unit, a highly specialized ICU where she was deeply skilled, deeply respected, and deeply embedded in the culture, the precepting relationship struggled. She went through the motions. She was competent and professional. But the energy was not there.

Then one day I did a pop-up visit while she was working in her preferred unit with an orientee.

What I found stopped me in the hallway.

She was not going through the motions. She was fully present, asking the orientee questions, going over documentation together, and conducting a deep clinical dive into the types of patients they treated in that unit and how the care differed from that in other areas. The depth of knowledge she was sharing was extraordinary. The investment was unmistakable.

A nurse walked by, glanced at them, and said without being asked: "I'm so glad you're the one training her."

Before I left that shift, I checked in with the orientee. She told me she had learned more that day than in any single shift of her orientation.

I shared that feedback with the preceptor. And then, because I had come to understand that this was not an RT who didn't want to precept, but an RT who precepted best when her environment matched her expertise and her identity, I asked her something I had been holding back.

I asked if I could place the preceptor badge on her.

She said yes. And as I pinned it on, she sang a little gospel song that I happen to know she loves.

That moment, the badge, the song, the joy, was not about a piece of plastic on a lanyard. It was about being seen accurately. About having someone understand not just what you can do, but the conditions under which you do it best. About being placed in an environment where your gifts are recognized, your expertise is respected, and your leadership emerges naturally because it has always been there, waiting for the right context to call it forward.

That is what intentional assignment does. And that is what the badge represents.

I got them for my preceptors because I wanted them to feel specialized. Because they are specialized. Because the work of guiding a new respiratory therapist through the most vulnerable transition of their professional life is not a side task or an administrative add-on. It is a distinct, skilled, important role that deserves to be named and visible.

What I did not fully anticipate was what would happen when the rest of the hospital noticed.

A new preceptor told me about the moment it clicked for her. She was walking through the unit when a nursing leader, someone from entirely outside the respiratory therapy department, glanced at her badge and acknowledged it. A small moment. A brief exchange. But the preceptor came back and told me about it with an energy I recognized immediately.

She felt set apart.

Not better than her colleagues. Not superior. Set apart in the specific way that comes from being seen in your role, from having the work you do recognized by someone who didn't have to notice, in a hallway where nobody was required to pay attention.

That moment cost nothing. And it changed how she saw herself as a preceptor.

This is not a small thing. Identity is one of the most powerful drivers of professional behavior, more powerful, in many cases, than incentives, instructions, or even skills training. A preceptor who sees themselves as someone who was handed an extra assignment will do the minimum required to complete it. A preceptor who sees themselves as a specialized educator, whose role is visible, recognized, and valued, will bring a fundamentally different level of investment to every shift they share with an orientee.

The badge is a symbol. But symbols, in the right culture, are extraordinarily powerful.

Precepting as a Clinical Ladder Requirement

The specialization is not only symbolic. It is structural. In our department, serving as a preceptor is a requirement for advancing on the clinical ladder.

This decision was intentional and important. It communicates that developing other respiratory therapists is not optional for clinicians who want to grow professionally. It is part of what growth means. An RT who advances on the clinical ladder is not just someone who has accumulated more clinical experience. They are someone who has demonstrated the ability and willingness to invest that experience in someone else.

That standard changes the culture around precepting in ways that nothing else quite replicates. When advancing professionally requires developing others, precepting stops being something that happens to willing volunteers and starts being something the entire department understands as part of professional excellence. It normalizes teaching as a core RT competency, not an extra, and creates a pipeline of preceptors motivated not just by goodwill but by genuine professional investment.

It also, not incidentally, makes the Preceptor Power Hours even more valuable, because preceptors now have a personal stake in developing the skills those sessions offer. The clinical ladder gives them a reason to take the badge seriously. The badge gives them an identity worth growing into. And the Power Hours give them the tools to do it well.

Together, those three things, recognition, structure, and development, create something most departments spend years trying to build and never quite achieve: a preceptor community that is proud of what it does, equipped to do it well, and motivated to keep getting better.

Let me tell you something practical that took me longer to figure out than I would like to admit.

Scheduling matters more than most educators realize.

I run my Preceptor Power Hours at 7:30 in the morning, during shift change, that narrow window when the night shift is wrapping up and the day shift is arriving. Both in person for those who are present and virtually for those who are not working but want to attend.

This timing is not accidental. It is strategic.

Shift change is one of the few moments in a respiratory therapy department when multiple people are naturally in the same space at the same time, without the full weight of a patient assignment bearing down on them yet. The night shift preceptors are present. The day shift preceptors are arriving. The window is brief, which creates a natural time boundary that keeps the session focused and respects everyone's time.

But here is the piece that makes the biggest difference, and I cannot overstate this:

My supervisors attend. My department manager attends.

Every single session. Without fail.

That decision, made early and maintained consistently, communicates something to every preceptor in that room that no facilitator's introduction or mission statement ever could. It says: *This is not something the educator invented because she needed a project. This is something leadership believes in enough to show up for. Your development matters to the people who run this department.*

That message changes the energy of the room. It changes the willingness of preceptors to engage honestly. It changes the perceived value of the time they are giving. And it changes the accountability, because when a preceptor knows that their manager has heard the same tools and frameworks they have, the expectation that those tools will be used becomes implicit and mutual.

If you take one logistical lesson from this chapter, let it be this: get your leadership in the room. Not occasionally. Every time.

The Buy-In Problem, and How to Solve It

I would be doing you a disservice if I described Preceptor Power Hours as something that preceptors immediately embrace with enthusiasm and gratitude. Some do. Many do not at first.

The resistance comes in familiar forms. *I'm too busy. Is this mandatory? I have a full assignment, can't I just get the notes?*

And my personal favorite, delivered with the particular energy of someone who has been in respiratory therapy long enough to have seen many initiatives come and go: *We tried something like this before and it didn't stick.*

These responses are not laziness or apathy. They are entirely reasonable reactions of people who are already stretched thin, who have learned from experience that not every well-intentioned program delivers on its promise, and who are protecting their most finite resource, time, until they have evidence that spending it here is worth it.

Your job, especially in the early sessions, is to provide that evidence.

Here is what I have found works:

Make the first session impossible to ignore. Choose a topic that every preceptor in your department is currently struggling with, not something theoretically important, but something that is causing friction right now. Boundaries and expectations in the orientation relationship is a perennial one, because it is something almost every preceptor navigates poorly at the beginning and nobody ever teaches them how to do well. When preceptors walk out of that first session with a specific, usable tool for something that has been quietly frustrating them, they tell other preceptors. Word travels.

Feed people. I am completely serious. Food at 7:30 in the morning is not a luxury. It is a buy-in strategy. A preceptor who might have talked themselves out of attending will often talk themselves into it when breakfast is involved. This is not bribery. It is hospitality.

And hospitality communicates welcome in a way that a calendar invite simply cannot.

Name the resistance out loud. In the first session, I acknowledge directly that some people in the room may be wondering whether this is worth their time. I tell them I respect that question. And then I make a commitment: every session will end with something they can use immediately, or I have not done my job. That promise, kept consistently, builds trust faster than anything else.

Let the converts do the selling. After a few sessions, you will have preceptors who are visibly energized by the work, who are applying the tools, who are having better orientee conversations, who are showing up early and staying late to keep the discussion going. Those people are your best recruitment asset. Their testimony carries more weight than anything you could say yourself.

The Topic That Fills Every Room

If I could only run one Preceptor Power Hour topic for the rest of my career, I know exactly which one I would choose.

Boundaries and expectations in the orientation relationship.

Every single time I have facilitated this session, the energy in the room shifts within the first ten minutes. Preceptors who came in quiet become vocal. Preceptors who seemed disengaged lean forward. Because this topic, the specific, practical, emotionally loaded question of how to establish clear expectations with a new orientee without coming across as cold, how to hold those boundaries when the orientee pushes against them, how to have the conversation when something is not working, is something every preceptor is navigating and almost none of them have been given tools to navigate well.

The conversations that surface in this session are some of the most honest I have ever facilitated. Preceptors talk about the orientee who texted them constantly on their days off. The one who became emotionally dependent in ways that felt inappropriate but were hard to name. The one who interpreted every piece of feedback as a personal attack. The one the preceptor genuinely liked as a person but was not sure would make it as a clinician, and the agony of holding both of those things at the same time.

These are not small problems. They are the problems that cause good preceptors to quietly ask not to be assigned an orientee again. And they are almost entirely preventable with the right tools and the right conversation at the beginning of the relationship.

The framework I teach in this session is simple enough to remember and specific enough to actually use. We call it the First Week Conversation, a structured, intentional discussion that happens in the first three days of every orientation, before the relationship has a chance to develop patterns that are hard to undo. It covers four things: how we will communicate; how I will give you feedback and how I need you to receive it; what I expect from you and what you can expect from me; and what we will do when something isn't working.

That last one, what we will do when something isn't working, is the part most preceptors skip, because naming the possibility of difficulty feels like inviting it.

What they discover, often with visible relief, is that naming it early actually prevents it. When both people know the plan before the crisis, the crisis is far less likely to become a relationship-ending event.

Sample Topics: A Full Year of Preceptor Power Hours

One of the practical challenges of running a monthly session is sustaining topic quality across twelve months. Here is a full year of topics that I have either run myself or developed for use in this context. Each one is specific enough to anchor a real discussion and relevant enough to generate genuine engagement.

Month 1: First Week Conversations, Setting Boundaries and Expectations That Stick. The foundation. Start here, every year, with every new cohort of preceptors. Even experienced preceptors benefit from revisiting this one.

Month 2: Teaching Clinical Reasoning, How to Share What's in Your Head. The think-aloud approach. How to narrate your reasoning in real time so the learner can see inside a clinical mind at work.

Month 3: Feedback That Builds, Delivering Hard Truths Without Breaking Trust. The session that generates the most emotional resonance. Most preceptors either over-soften or over-deliver. This session finds the middle.

Month 4: The Struggling Orientee, How to Know, What to Do, When to Escalate. One of the most anxiety-producing situations a preceptor faces. This session gives them a framework for early identification and a clear path forward.

Month 5: When to Step In and When to Step Back, The Art of Productive Struggle. The Protector's dilemma. How to let a learner struggle in ways that build rather than break, and how to know the difference.

Month 6: Mid-Year Check-In, What's Working, What Isn't, What Do You Need? Not a topic session but a community session. Take the temperature. Celebrate wins. Address patterns. Let preceptors hear from each other.

Month 7: The Emotional Side of Precepting, Compassion Fatigue, Burnout, and Boundaries. The session nobody runs but everybody needs. Precepting is emotionally demanding work. Naming that out loud in a supported space matters.

Month 8: Teaching Across Differences, Generational, Cultural, and Learning Style Gaps. Practical strategies for preceptors who are struggling to connect with an orientee whose learning style or background is very different from their own.

Month 9: Documentation and Communication, What to Write, What to Say, and When. The practical mechanics of orientation documentation, how to write objective, useful feedback and how to communicate concerns to the educator and leadership.

Month 10: Building Confidence Without Inflating It, The Fine Line. How to develop a new RT's sense of competence authentically, neither falsely reassuring them nor inadvertently undermining them.

Month 11: After Orientation, What Happens Next and How Preceptors Can Stay Involved. The transition from orientation to independent practice. How preceptors can continue to support their orientees informally after the formal relationship ends.

Month 12: Celebration and Reflection, What We Built This Year. End the year with intentional recognition. Name the preceptors who showed up, grew, and made a difference. Celebrate the orientees who thrived. Look forward to what's next.

What Preceptors Actually Need to Hear

Preceptors need to hear that what they do is hard.

Not in a commiserating, isn't-it-awful way. In a genuine, clear-eyed, I-see-you way. They carry a patient assignment and a teaching relationship simultaneously. They navigate the emotional complexity of being responsible for someone else's professional development while managing their own. They give feedback that is sometimes received badly. They invest in orientees who sometimes leave anyway. They show up, shift after shift, doing a job that nobody formally trained them for, and they do it largely without acknowledgment.

Your Preceptor Power Hour is not just a skill development session. It is an act of recognition. Every time you gather your preceptors in that room, at 7:30 in the morning, with coffee and food and leadership present and a topic that actually matters, you are telling them: I see what you do. I know it is hard. You are not alone in it. And you deserve to be developed just as much as the people you are developing.

That message, delivered consistently over time, does something remarkable. It turns preceptors into believers. It turns believers into advocates. And it turns advocates into the kind of educators who will one day pull a colleague aside in a hallway and hold her accountable, warmly, confidently, and with just enough humor, using the tools she taught them.

That is the chin check. And that is everything.

Chapter Summary

- Preceptor Power Hours are monthly, sixty-minute structured sessions designed specifically for active preceptors, not all staff, not new RTs, but the people currently doing the teaching.
- Preceptor identity matters as much as preceptor skill. Visible recognition, a badge, a title, a moment of acknowledgment from a colleague in a hallway, builds the professional identity that drives investment in the role.
- Tying preceptor development to clinical ladder advancement communicates that developing others is not optional for professional growth. It is part of what growth means in this department.
- A tiered preceptor system, four tiers based on experience, clinical area, and teaching readiness, ensures that the right preceptor is matched with the right orientee every time. Preceptors choose

their tier; supervisors and the educator approve placements.

- Intentional assignment matching, by personality, learning style, and preceptor capacity, creates the conditions where learning is most likely to happen and burnout is most effectively prevented.
- Daily two-way evaluations, reviewed by the educator, give real-time visibility into every orientation relationship, allowing issues to be identified and addressed before they become crises.
- The goal of every session is threefold: equip preceptors with practical tools, create space for honest conversation about the challenges of precepting, and build a community so preceptors feel connected rather than isolated.
- Scheduling at shift change, with leadership present every session, communicates that preceptor development is a departmental priority, not an educator's side project.
- Buy-in is earned, not assumed. Choose an immediately relevant first topic, provide food, name the resistance directly, and let the converts do the selling.
- The topic that generates the most energy and the most immediate impact: setting boundaries and expectations in the first week of the orientation relationship.

- A full year of monthly topics is provided in this chapter, specific, practical, and ready to use.
- Preceptors need to be developed just as intentionally as the RTs they are developing. Preceptor Power Hours are how you do that.

Reflection Prompts

1. Who are your active preceptors right now? When was the last time someone asked them how the precepting relationship was going for them, not just for the orientee?
2. If you were to tier your preceptors today based on experience, teaching readiness, and the populations they work best with, what would that look like? Who would be in each tier? Who is ready to move up?
3. How are preceptor assignments currently made in your department? Is personality matching part of the process, or is assignment purely logistical? What would change if it weren't?
4. Does feedback in your department flow in both directions during orientation? If not, what would it take to implement a simple daily two-way evaluation process?
5. Is your department leadership present for preceptor development conversations? If not, what would it take to get them in the room?
6. Think about the preceptor in your department who is doing the most important quiet work,

showing up, investing, growing. Have you told them lately what their contribution means?

The First Week Conversation: A Starter Framework

Use this as a discussion anchor in your first Preceptor Power Hour session on boundaries and expectations. Ask preceptors to review it, react to it, and adapt it to their own voice.

Opening: "Before we get into the clinical work, I want to take a few minutes to talk about how we are going to work together. I want this orientation to go well for both of us, and in my experience, the relationships that go best are the ones where we are both clear from the beginning about what to expect."

Communication: "Here is how I prefer to communicate outside of our shifts together, and here is what I need from you in terms of response time and availability. My days off are my days off. I want to support you, and I also need to be able to recharge. Let's talk about what that looks like."

Feedback: "I am going to give you feedback regularly, some of it positive, some of it developmental. I am going to try to be specific and timely. What I need from you is to receive it as information, not judgment. If a piece of feedback lands hard, tell me. We can talk about it. What I cannot do is soften it to the point where it stops being useful."

Expectations: "Here is what I expect from you during this orientation. Here is what you can expect from me. Let's make sure we are both clear, and let's agree to check in on these expectations at the midpoint of orientation, not just at the end."

When Things Aren't Working: "If something isn't working between us, if you feel like your needs aren't being met, or if I feel like the orientation isn't progressing the way it should, I want us to be able to say that directly, to each other, before it becomes a bigger problem. Can we agree to that?"

Coming Up in Chapter Nine

We have built the foundation of preceptor development. In Chapter Nine, we zoom out to the broader question of leadership development across the entire department: how to grow RT leaders at every level, how to identify potential before it announces itself, and how to create the kind of intentional leadership pipeline that keeps your best people engaged, growing, and invested in the future of the profession they chose.

"Developing preceptors is not optional.
It is the lever that moves everything else."

09

GROWING THE NEXT GENERATION OF RT LEADERS

Intentional Development vs. Accidental Leadership

"The growth and development of people is the highest calling of leadership."
– Harvey S. Firestone

Three Preceptors. Same Mistake. One Honest Orientee.

She was in her second week of orientation.

I was doing a routine check-in, the kind I do with every new orientee early in the process, not to evaluate but to listen. How are things going? How is your confidence level? What is feeling comfortable, and what is not?

She told me things were going well. Her preceptors were excellent. She felt supported. And then she paused, chose her words carefully, and told me the truth.

She felt uncertain during rapid responses. Uncomfortable. Overwhelmed. Not because she didn't care or wasn't trying, but because she genuinely did not yet know what to do. And standing at a bedside during a rapid response, surrounded by urgency and expectation, with a preceptor nearby who was clearly waiting for her to act, that gap between what was expected and what she was capable of had been happening repeatedly.

“Three times,” she said. With three different preceptors.

I asked her what she thought the solution was.

What happened next is the moment I want you to sit with.

This new graduate, two weeks into her first job, still learning what normal looks like, still building the clinical vocabulary that will eventually become second nature, looked at me and articulated, clearly and specifically, exactly what she needed.

"I think the solution would be if I attended rapid responses after I've gone through ICU orientation and had more time to develop my critical thinking skills. Maybe after orientation, go back to the general care areas first, and then attend rapid responses."

She knew. She had diagnosed her own learning gap, identified the sequencing problem, and proposed a developmentally appropriate solution, all in a second-week check-in conversation that most orientation programs never have.

I asked her what her preceptors had been doing during these rapid responses. She said they were there, they were answering her questions, they were trying to give her time to make decisions and learn how to respond.

And there it was.

Three experienced, well-intentioned preceptors had made the same mistake. They had given a new graduate space to make decisions during a rapid response, because that is what good preceptors do for developing clinicians. Productive struggle. Room to grow. Autonomy that builds confidence.

Except this was a new graduate in her second week of orientation, still learning what normal looks like. She had not yet developed the clinical thinking skills that productive struggle requires as its foundation. Giving her space to make decisions she was not yet equipped to make was not developmental autonomy. It was, however unintentionally, abandonment.

What she needed, what every new graduate needs in that moment, was the opposite. She needed her preceptor at the bedside, making the decision, narrating the reasoning out loud, and debriefing with her afterward. Not "your turn" but "watch me, here's why, now let's talk about what you saw."

Three preceptors. Same mistake. Not because any of them were wrong about the value of autonomy in learning; they weren't. But because none of them had been given the specific guidance that distinguishes developmental autonomy from premature independence. The guidance that says: *The level of challenge you offer must match the level of development your learner has actually reached, not the level you hope they're at.*

That conversation with one honest orientee became the topic of our next Preceptor Power Hour.

That is what intentional leadership development looks like. Not waiting for problems to become crises. Building the feedback loops, the check-ins, and the psychological safety that surface them early, and then using what surfaces to make the whole system smarter.

Accidental Leadership vs. Intentional Development

Most respiratory therapy departments develop leaders accidentally.

Not negligently. Not carelessly. Accidentally, meaning that leadership development happens as a byproduct of other things rather than as a deliberate, designed process. An RT gets a charge assignment because the schedule needed filling. Another gets asked to precept because they were available. A third ends up on a committee because nobody else volunteered. Over time, some of these accidental assignments produce genuine leaders, people who discover capabilities they didn't know they had because a situation demanded it.

But accidental leadership development has a significant problem: it is neither equitable, efficient, nor reliable.

It is not equitable because accidental opportunities go to the people who are most visible, most available, and most similar to the people making the assignments, meaning that quieter RTs, newer RTs, and RTs whose potential does not announce itself loudly are systematically overlooked. The leadership pipeline that emerges from accidental development reflects not the full range of talent in the department but the narrow range that happened to be in the right place at the right time.

It is not efficient because it wastes time. An RT who is ready for a leadership challenge at year two but doesn't receive one until year five has lost three years of development, and the department has lost three years of the contribution that development would have produced.

And it is not reliable because it depends on luck. The right supervisor noticing. The right opportunity opening up. The right colleague choosing to invest. When leadership development is left to chance, it produces inconsistent results, some extraordinary leaders who were fortunate enough to encounter the right conditions, and a much larger number of capable RTs who never fully became what they were capable of being because nobody deliberately created the conditions for it.

Intentional leadership development changes all of that. It is not complicated. It does not require a formal program or a significant budget. It requires an educator, and a department culture, that treats leadership capacity as something to be actively cultivated in every RT, at every level, starting on day one. Here is how.

Assign, Don't Wait

The single most powerful thing you can do to develop leaders in your department is also the simplest:

Give people things to do before they feel ready.

Not irresponsibly. Not without support. But deliberately, with intention, slightly ahead of where they currently are, because that is where growth lives. Not in the comfortable repetition of things already mastered, but in the productive stretch of being asked to do something that requires becoming a little more than you currently are.

The RT who has never charged a unit will not feel ready the first time you ask them to. The one who has never led a huddle will stumble through the first one. The new graduate who has never taught a family member how to use a home nebulizer will be uncertain and imperfect and will learn more from that fifteen-minute conversation than from three competency modules on the same topic.

This is not sink-or-swim. Sink-or-swim is assigning the challenge and walking away. Intentional stretch assignment is assigning the challenge, staying close enough to catch what needs catching, and debriefing afterward with the specific question: "What did you learn about yourself in that moment?"

The difference between those two approaches is the difference between an experience that builds and one that breaks. Both involve difficulty. Only one involves development.

In practice, assign leadership reps early and often:

Ask a new RT, in their first month, to lead the post-treatment assessment debrief with their preceptor. Not to make decisions alone, but to practice organizing and presenting clinical information out loud.

Ask a second-year RT to host one station at the next Level Up Week. Not because they are the most expert in the room, but because teaching something is the fastest way to understand it more deeply.

Ask the RT who always has opinions in the break room to bring one of those opinions to a staff meeting, formally, with a proposal. Not to guarantee the idea will be adopted, but to build the habit of turning observation into advocacy.

Ask the charge therapist who has been informally mentoring new graduates for years to formalize that relationship, to become a Tier Two preceptor, to attend Preceptor Power Hours, to have their contribution named and recognized as what it is.

Every one of these assignments is a leadership rep. And leadership, like clinical skill, develops through repetition, through the accumulation of small, supported challenges that build capacity over time.

The Ownership Shift: Involving Staff in Decisions

I want to tell you about a workflow change that cost nothing and changed everything.

A staff RT, experienced, competent, and quietly disengaged in the way that some experienced staff become when they have been doing the same job in the same place for long enough to stop expecting things to change, mentioned something in passing during a shift. A frustration about a scheduling pattern that was creating inefficiency and, more importantly, was affecting patient care during transitions.

It was the kind of comment that gets made and forgotten in most departments. A complaint offered into the air, not quite directed at anyone, not quite expecting a response.

I asked her to tell me more.

And then I asked her a question that I have found, over years of practice, to be one of the most powerful leadership development interventions available to any educator or manager:

"What would you do if it were your decision to make?"

She paused. Because nobody had asked her that before. And then she answered, thoughtfully, specifically, with the kind of operational detail that only comes from someone who has been living inside the problem long enough to understand it from the inside out.

We implemented her suggestion. Not a version of it. Not a modified, committee-approved, administratively diluted version. Her suggestion, as she described it, with her name attached to it in the communication to the department.

What happened next was not subtle.

She started bringing more ideas. Not complaints, ideas. Specific, considered, solution-oriented contributions to department conversations that she had previously observed from a distance. Her attitude toward the department shifted in ways that were visible to everyone around her. The ownership she felt over one scheduling change gradually expanded into a broader sense of ownership over the department itself. This was no longer just a place she worked. It was a place she had helped shape.

This is the ownership shift. And it does not happen through team-building exercises, engagement surveys, or motivational posters in the break room. It happens when someone in authority looks at a staff member and communicates, through action, not just words, "Your perspective matters here. Your ideas have weight. This department is better because you are thinking about it."

That message, delivered consistently and backed by genuine follow-through, is one of the most powerful retention and leadership development tools available to any department. It costs nothing except the willingness to listen and the courage to act on what you hear.

Structured Mentorship Pairs: Building the Relationship That Builds the Leader

Mentorship in most respiratory therapy departments is accidental. It happens when a newer RT is fortunate enough to work alongside a more experienced one who is generous with their time and wisdom. It is informal, unstructured, and entirely dependent on the chemistry of the relationship and the availability of the people involved.

This produces some extraordinary mentorship relationships. It also produces enormous inequity, because the new RT whose personality naturally connects with a senior colleague's gets something that the quieter, more reserved new RT working different shifts never receives.

Structured mentorship pairs change that.

A structured mentorship pair is an intentional match, made by the educator, with input from supervisors, between a developing RT and a more experienced one, with a specific developmental purpose and a minimum commitment of a thirty-minute conversation each month. Not about patients. Not about tasks. About the developing RT's goals, growth edges, and professional trajectory.

The conversations are guided by three questions that I have found, over time, to be reliably productive:

"What is energizing you right now, in your work, in your development, in your professional life?"

"What is frustrating or challenging you, and what do you think is underneath that?"

"What do you want to be able to do, know, or become in the next six months that you can't do, don't know, or aren't yet?"

These questions do something that performance reviews and competency check-ins never do: they treat the developing RT as a whole person with a professional trajectory that belongs to them, not as a skill set to be verified or a gap to be remediated. They communicate that the organization is interested not just in what the RT can do today but in who they are becoming.

The mentor's role in these conversations is not to advise, direct, or solve. It is to listen, to reflect back, to ask the next question. The most effective mentors I have seen are not the ones with the most answers. They are the ones who ask the questions that help the developing RT find their own.

Safe Failure: The Leadership Laboratory

Leaders are not developed in the absence of failure. They are developed in environments where failure is processed rather than punished, where the question after something goes wrong is not "who is responsible?" but "what did we learn, and what do we do differently?"

This is harder to build than it sounds. Healthcare is a high-stakes environment with a deep cultural history of blame, of individual accountability that slides easily into individual shame. The RT who makes an error, documents it honestly, and brings it forward for discussion is taking a professional risk in most departments. The RT who quietly covers the gap and moves on is taking a human one.

Safe failure is not the absence of accountability. It is the presence of psychological safety alongside accountability, the environment in which an RT can say "I tried something, it didn't work, here is what I learned" and be met with genuine engagement rather than judgment.

Building this environment requires consistent, visible modeling from leadership. It requires the educator who shares their own mistakes in Preceptor Power Hours. The supervisor who responds to an error report with curiosity before criticism. The charge therapist who debriefs a difficult rapid response by asking "what would we do differently?" rather than "who dropped the ball?"

It also requires celebrating the attempts, not just the successes. The RT who proposed a workflow change that didn't work out needs to hear, specifically and publicly, that the act of proposing it was valuable, that departments get better through the accumulation of ideas, including those that don't pan out. That the RT who tries and fails has contributed more to the department's development than the RT who never tries at all.

When that message is delivered consistently, in staff meetings, in huddles, in individual conversations, it produces something remarkable: a department full of RTs who are willing to lead. Who are willing to propose, to try, to speak up, to take the professional risk of being wrong in front of their colleagues because the culture has demonstrated, repeatedly, that being wrong is not the worst thing that can happen here.

Giving up on trying is.

The One Question That Changes Everything

I want to close this chapter with the simplest and most powerful leadership development tool I know. It costs nothing. It takes less than five minutes. And it has the potential to change the professional trajectory of every RT who hears it asked with genuine intent.

"Where do you want to go?"

Not as a performance review question. Not as part of an annual goal-setting form. As a real question, asked in a real conversation, by someone who is genuinely prepared to listen to the answer and do something with it.

Most RTs have never been asked this question. Not really. They have been asked whether their competencies are current, whether they are meeting performance standards, and whether they have any concerns about their assignment. They have not been asked by someone with the authority and the intention to help where they want their career to go or what the department could do to help them get there.

The absence of that question communicates something: that the organization's interest in the RT is limited to their current performance, that what matters is what they can do today, not what they might become tomorrow. That message, absorbed over months and years, produces exactly the disengagement and departure that every department is trying to prevent.

The presence of the question communicates something entirely different. It communicates: *You have a future here, and we are interested in it. Your ambition is welcome. Your goals matter. You are not just a body filling a shift; you are a person becoming something, and we want to be part of that becoming.*

That message, delivered in a five-minute conversation, followed by genuine follow-through, is one of the most powerful retention and leadership development interventions available to any educator. It does not require a program. It does not require a budget. It requires presence, intention, and the willingness to ask the question and mean it.

Ask it this week. For every RT on your team who has never heard it.

And then listen, really listen, to what they tell you.

Because the answer to "where do you want to go?" is also the answer to "how do I keep this person?" And "what does this department need to become?" And "who is the next generation of RT leaders standing right in front of me, waiting to be asked?"

They are waiting. Ask.

Chapter Summary

- Most departments develop leaders accidentally, through proximity, availability, and circumstance rather than intentional design. Accidental leadership development is inequitable, inefficient, and unreliable.
- Intentional leadership development begins with stretch assignments, giving RTs leadership responsibilities slightly ahead of where they currently are, with support and a structured debrief to make the challenge developmental rather than overwhelming.
- The ownership shift happens when staff are genuinely involved in decisions, not consulted and then overridden, but heard, acted upon, and credited. One idea implemented changes how an RT relates to their entire department.
- Structured mentorship pairs, intentionally matched monthly and guided by three specific questions, provide the developmental

conversation that accidental mentorship cannot reliably deliver.

- Safe failure is not the absence of accountability. It is the presence of psychological safety alongside it, an environment where trying and learning is celebrated even when the attempt doesn't succeed.
- The one question that changes everything: "Where do you want to go?" Asked genuinely and followed through intentionally, it is one of the most powerful leadership development and retention tools available to any educator.

Reflection Prompts

1. Think about the last leadership opportunity that opened up in your department. How was it filled, intentionally or accidentally? Who might have been ready for it that nobody considered?
2. When was the last time a staff RT's suggestion directly changed something in your department and they knew it? What did that do to their engagement?
3. Who on your team needs a stretch assignment right now? What would you give them, and what support would you put in place to make it developmental rather than overwhelming?
4. When did you last ask a staff RT where they want to go, genuinely, with the intention of helping them get there? What did they tell you, or what might they tell you if you asked?

Coming Up in Chapter Ten

We have built the LEAD pillar, from the philosophy of leadership without a title to the practical strategies that develop leaders intentionally across every level of the department. In Chapter Ten, we turn to the final pillar: Stay. Not retention as a metric. Not retention as a perk program. Retention as a culture, built shift by shift, conversation by conversation, in the environment that either earns people's commitment or quietly loses it.

*"The answer to 'where do you want to go?'
is also the answer to 'how do I keep this person?' They are waiting to be asked."*

10

WHAT STAY ACTUALLY REQUIRES

"People don't stay because of what you pay them.
They stay because of what you make them feel,
about their work, about their future, and about themselves."

A Question Before We Begin

Before you read another word of this chapter, I want you to sit with one question.

Not answer it out loud. Not write it down. Just sit with it, honestly, without the professional instinct to optimize or deflect.

If your best respiratory therapist received a call tomorrow from another department offering them a new opportunity, what would make them stay?

Not what you hope would make them stay. Not what your retention policy says should make them stay. What would actually make them stay, based on what you know about that person, what they need, what they have told you directly or indirectly about what is missing, and what the honest state of your department's culture would offer them in that moment of decision?

Take a moment with that question. Because your answer, whatever it is, is the real subject of this chapter.

The Plateau Nobody Talks About

I want to tell you about a season of my own career that I have not described in detail until now.

It was not the COVID exhaustion I wrote about in the Introduction; that came later and was its own particular kind of breaking. This was quieter. More insidious, in some ways, because it did not feel like a crisis. It felt like fine.

I was mid-career. Competent, deeply, reliably competent. I knew my clinical work well. I showed up. I performed. I was, by every external measure, exactly what a solid respiratory therapist looks like. I had moved through roles: staff RT, lead therapist, supervisor, manager, and somewhere in that progression, in the accumulation of titles, responsibilities, and years, I had stopped expecting the next thing.

Not because I had given up. But because nobody had shown me that a "next thing" existed.

The ladder I could see had ended. Not dramatically; it had not been pulled away or blocked. It had simply stopped appearing in front of me. The path forward that had once felt like a natural progression had, somewhere in the middle years, become a plateau. And plateaus, when you are standing on them long enough, start to feel like destinations.

I was good at my job. I told myself that was enough. And in the quiet, private way that competent people talk themselves into settling, I started to believe it.

What I did not know, could not see from where I was standing, was that the plateau was not the end of the path. It was a landing where someone should have met me with a map.

Nobody did. Not because nobody cared. But because in most departments, nobody is watching for the mid-career plateau. The systems we build for development, the onboarding processes, the orientation structures, the new graduate residency programs are designed for the beginning of a career. The RT who has been there five years, who is competent and reliable and no longer requires active management, tends to disappear entirely from the developmental conversation.

And in disappearing from the conversation, they disappear slowly, quietly, and, often invisibly, from the department.

I didn't leave. I found my path forward, through the friend who made the phone call, through the educator role that changed everything, through the discovery that the plateau had never been a destination at all. But I think about the RTs who didn't find it. The ones who stood on that same plateau, looked around, saw no map, and made the entirely rational decision to look for one somewhere else.

They did not leave because they didn't care about the work. They left because the work stopped having a visible future.

That is what this chapter is about. Not retention as a crisis to be managed, but growth as a culture to be built, one that makes the future visible for every RT in your department, at every stage of their career, before they start looking for it somewhere else.

Why Growth Is the Most Underestimated Retention Factor

Ask most department leaders what drives RT turnover and you will hear a familiar list. Scheduling. Burnout. Compensation. The travel therapy market. Generational differences in workforce expectations. These are real factors. They deserve real attention.

But here is what the data, and more importantly, the honest conversations, consistently reveal: the factor that most reliably predicts whether a good RT stays or goes is not on that list.

It is whether they can see where they are going.

Not whether the path is easy. Not whether it is fast. Whether it exists, visibly, specifically, in a form that connects who they are today to who they could become if they stay.

Research on employee retention across healthcare consistently identifies a lack of growth opportunity as one of the top drivers of voluntary turnover, ranking above compensation in most studies when controlling for extreme pay disparities. Amy Wrzesniewski's research on work orientation found that employees who experience their work as a calling, as something connected to personal growth, meaning, and identity, demonstrate dramatically higher retention and engagement than those who experience it as a job or even a career. And in respiratory therapy specifically, AARC workforce data repeatedly surfaces professional development opportunities as a top factor in both retention and job satisfaction.

The implication is clear: RTs who are growing stay. RTs who have stopped growing, or who cannot see how they will grow, leave. And the departments that retain their best people are not necessarily the ones with the best pay or the best schedules. They are the ones that have figured out how to make growth visible, ongoing, and personally meaningful for every RT they employ.

This is not complicated in theory. It is demanding in practice because making growth visible requires knowing each person well enough to understand what growth means to them specifically. Not what the clinical ladder says growth looks like. With this history, these ambitions, and this particular set of gifts, what this RT needs to see in front of them to believe that staying is worth it.

That kind of knowing requires relationship. And relationship requires investment. And investment, the kind that actually changes retention outcomes, looks like the three things we are about to discuss.

A Clinical Ladder That Actually Means Something

Most respiratory therapy departments have a clinical ladder. Many of those ladders are, to put it charitably, decorative.

They exist. They have levels, criteria, and perhaps a modest compensation differential between tiers. They are mentioned during onboarding and referenced occasionally in performance reviews. And they have almost no meaningful impact on how RTs experience their professional development, because they were designed to recognize achievement rather than to create it. They describe where an RT has arrived, not where they are going.

A clinical ladder that actually means something does the opposite. It is not a recognition system. It is a development roadmap: a visible, specific, personally meaningful map that shows every RT in the department exactly where they could go from where they are right now, what it would take to get there, and the support the department will provide along the way.

The difference between those two things is the difference between a plaque on a wall and a conversation that changes someone's professional trajectory.

Here is what a meaningful clinical ladder includes:

Specific, achievable criteria that describe behaviors and contributions rather than just credentials and years of service. Not "five years of experience and RRT-NPS" but "demonstrates consistent clinical leadership in complex patient populations, serves as a Tier Three or Four preceptor, and has led or contributed to at least one department improvement initiative."

A development pathway, not just a description of where you need to be, but a concrete plan for how to get there. What certifications does the department support financially? What preceptor tier should this RT be working toward? What committee involvement, quality improvement project, or leadership development experience would move them forward?

Regular, unhurried review conversations, not annual performance evaluations, but quarterly or semi-annual developmental check-ins specifically focused on the clinical ladder. Where are you? Where do you want to go? What has happened since we last talked, and what do you need next?

Genuine organizational support, meaning the department actually funds certifications, actually accommodates study time, actually celebrates advancement publicly and specifically. A clinical ladder that exists on paper but receives no organizational investment communicates that the organization does not take it seriously. And neither will the staff.

When a clinical ladder has all of these elements, when it is a living document rather than a static one, a conversation rather than a form, a genuine organizational commitment rather than a checkbox, it does something powerful. It gives every RT in the department a reason to think about next year instead of just next week. It makes the future visible. And visible futures are worth staying for.

Career Conversations That Happen Before the Exit Interview

The most important retention conversation in any department is not the exit interview.

It is the conversation that happens six months before someone starts thinking about leaving, when they are still engaged enough to be influenced, still invested enough to be reached, still present enough to hear that the department sees their potential and is prepared to do something about it.

Most departments have the exit interview. Very few have the proactive career conversation.

Here is what a proactive career conversation looks like in practice.

It is scheduled, not reactive, not triggered by a concern, but built into the rhythm of the year as a regular touchpoint for every staff RT. Quarterly for new graduates and early-career staff. Semi-annually for mid-career staff. Annually for experienced staff, supplemented by the informal check-ins that happen in hallways and break rooms throughout the year.

It is focused specifically on the RT's professional trajectory, not on performance management or operational concerns. Those conversations have their own time and their own format. This conversation is for one thing: understanding where this person wants to go and what the department can do to help them get there.

It asks specific questions:

"What has energized you most in the last six months, clinically, professionally, personally?"

"What has been most frustrating or draining, and what do you think is underneath that?"

"Where do you want to be in your career two years from now? Five years?"

"What would you need to see from this department, specifically, to believe that staying is worth it?"

That last question is the hardest to ask. It requires vulnerability from the leader and honesty from the RT. It risks surfacing needs the department cannot meet, frustrations that have been building unaddressed, and ambitions that will require genuine organizational investment to support.

Ask it anyway.

Because the alternative, the exit interview, where a departing RT finally says what they needed two years ago and the department can do nothing with it, is infinitely more costly. In time. In money. In the loss of someone who might have stayed if someone had simply asked, in time to matter, what they needed to stay.

The proactive career conversation is not a guarantee of retention. Some RTs will tell you what they need and the department will not be able to provide it, and they will leave anyway, which is their right and sometimes the right outcome. But many will tell you something the department can address. Something that, addressed with genuine follow-through, changes the calculation entirely.

I stayed because someone asked what I needed before I had already decided to go.

That is a sentence worth building a practice around.

Specialty Tracks and Certification Support: The Signal That Changes Everything

There is a specific organizational behavior that communicates investment in an RT's future more clearly than almost anything else a department can do.

Paying for their certification.

Not because certifications are the point; they are not, in themselves, what retain people. But because the decision to invest financially in an RT's professional development sends a signal that transcends the dollar amount. It says: *We are betting on your future here. We believe you are worth developing. We are putting organizational resources behind that belief.*

That signal matters enormously, particularly to the mid-career RT who has been wondering, in the quiet way that mid-career plateaus produce, whether the department sees them as a long-term investment or a short-term resource.

Specialty certifications in respiratory therapy, such as RRT-ACCS, RRT-NPS, RRT-SDS, CPFT, and others, represent not just clinical expertise but also professional identity. The RT who holds an ACCS is not just more knowledgeable about critical care. They are someone whose specialized expertise has been formally recognized by the national credentialing body and, when the department supports the pursuit, by the organization they work for.

Beyond individual certifications, specialty tracks, and structured pathways that connect clinical experience, certification pursuit, preceptor development, and leadership involvement into a coherent professional trajectory give RTs something even more powerful than a credential. They give them a narrative. A story about their own professional development that has a direction, a purpose, and a destination worth working toward.

Building specialty tracks does not require a large budget or an elaborate program. It requires sitting down with each RT and asking: "What area of respiratory therapy do you want to go deep in? And what would a path toward becoming truly specialized in that area look like for you here?"

The answer to that question is a specialty track. And the department's willingness to walk that path alongside the RT, with support, with investment, with recognition at each milestone, is what transforms a clinical job into a professional home worth keeping.

The Five Things That Make RTs Stay

Growth is the most underestimated retention factor. But it does not stand alone. Here, briefly and honestly, are the five things that the research and the hallway conversations consistently identify as what actually makes respiratory therapists stay:

Growth. A visible, personally meaningful path forward that keeps the future interesting. We have spent this chapter on this one because it deserves it.

Belonging. The felt sense of being part of something that knows your name. Not just your assignment. You. The department that notices when you are having a hard week, that celebrates your wins specifically and publicly, that makes you feel like your presence matters beyond your productivity.

Purpose. The connection between the daily work and something larger than the shift. The RT who understands that what they do changes outcomes, for patients, for families, for the next generation of clinicians they develop, is the RT who finds meaning in the hard days as well as the good ones.

Being known. Having at least one person in the department, an educator, a supervisor, a colleague, who sees you as a whole person with a life and a history and a future, not just a skilled pair of hands filling a schedule. This is the simplest and most powerful retention factor I know. People stay where they feel seen.

Psychological safety. The ability to speak up, make mistakes, ask questions, and try new things without fear of judgment or retaliation. We have built this throughout the book, in the clinical reasoning culture, in preceptor relationships, and in department conversations. Here, in the context of retention, it is worth naming explicitly: RTs who do not feel safe to be imperfect leave. Quietly, usually. But reliably.

None of these five things require a budget line. All of them require intention. And all of them are available to every educator and department leader reading this, starting with the next shift, the next conversation, the next moment when a respiratory therapist in your department needs to feel that staying is worth it.

What Stay Requires: The Honest Summary

Retention is not a program. It is not a perk. It is not a sign-on bonus, a scheduling accommodation, or an annual engagement survey with a color-coded dashboard.

Retention is a culture. And cultures are built in the small, daily, accumulated choices of the people who lead, in hallways and break rooms, in five-minute conversations and moments of recognition that nobody scheduled and everybody remembered.

It is built when you ask the question before someone starts thinking about leaving.

It is built when you invest in someone's certification because you are betting on their future here.

It is built when a new graduate sees a clinical ladder that has steps they can actually climb toward something they actually want.

It is built when an experienced RT brings an idea to life and feels, perhaps for the first time in years, that this department is partly theirs.

It is built when someone who has been standing on a plateau looks up and sees, for the first time, that there is more path ahead of them. That the plateau was never the destination. That someone in this department noticed they had stopped climbing and decided to show them the way forward.

That is what stay requires.

Not more money. Not better parking. Not a bigger break room.

A visible future. A felt sense of belonging. The knowledge that someone here knows your name, sees your potential, and is invested, genuinely, specifically, with follow-through, in what you become.

Give your RTs that. And then watch what they give back.

Chapter Summary

- Growth is the most underestimated retention factor in respiratory therapy. RTs who can see a visible, meaningful path forward stay. RTs who cannot, regardless of how competent and committed they are, eventually leave.
- The mid-career plateau is the silent epidemic of RT retention. Developmental systems designed for new hires leave experienced staff invisible, and invisible staff become mobile staff.
- A clinical ladder that actually means something is a development roadmap, not a recognition system. It describes where an RT can go, what it takes to get there, and what the department will do to support the journey.

- Proactive career conversations, scheduled, focused, and asking the hard questions before someone starts thinking about leaving, are the most cost-effective retention intervention available to any department.
- Certification support and specialty tracks signal organizational investment in an RT's future. That signal changes how an RT understands their relationship with the department, from employee to invested professional.
- The five things that actually make RTs stay: growth, belonging, purpose, being known, and psychological safety. None require a budget. All require intention.

Reflection Prompts

1. Think about your most experienced staff RT, the one who has been there longest and whose departure would hurt the most. When was the last time you had a genuine career conversation with them? What do you think they would say if you asked what they need to stay?
2. Does your department's clinical ladder function as a development roadmap or a recognition system? What would it take to make it the former?
3. Who in your department is currently standing on a mid-career plateau, competent, reliable, and quietly invisible in the developmental conversation? What would showing them the next step look like?

4. When was the last time your department invested financially in an RT's professional development, certification, conference attendance, or specialty training? What signal did that send?

Coming Up in Chapter Eleven

We have established what Stay actually requires: growth, belonging, purpose, being known, and psychological safety. In Chapter Eleven, we go deeper into the most practical of these: visible career pathways. What does it actually look like to build a clinical ladder that RTs believe in, a specialty track that keeps ambitious clinicians engaged, and a career conversation practice that surfaces needs before they become departures?

"Retention is not a program.
It is a culture, built in the small, daily, accumulated choices of the people who lead."

11

THE EDUCATOR AS CULTURE KEEPER

"Culture is not what you say you value.
It is what people experience when they walk through your door, and whether they come back."

The Moment I Understood My Real Job

There is a version of the clinical educator role that lives entirely inside formal education moments.

Orientation schedules. Competency verification. Preceptor assignments. Skills checklists. New hire onboarding timelines. These are the things that appear on the job description, that get tracked in spreadsheets, that produce the documentation a department needs to demonstrate that its education program is functioning.

I was good at all of those things. I took them seriously. I still do.

But somewhere in the early months of my role (in the accumulation of interactions that happened outside scheduled education moments, in the hallways and break rooms, and during the quick conversations before shift change), I began to understand something that no job description had prepared me for.

What I did outside of formal education moments mattered more than what I did inside them.

Not because the formal moments weren't important. They were. But because the formal moments happen in a context, a department culture, that either amplifies or undermines everything the formal education process is trying to build. You can design the most thoughtful orientation program in the history of respiratory therapy. You can develop the most skilled preceptors, the most reflective clinical reasoning tools, the most intentional leadership development pathway. And if the culture that a new RT walks into every shift communicates that questions are burdensome, that mistakes are shameful, that growth is accidental and recognition is rare, the formal program will fight that culture every day and lose.

Culture is not the backdrop of education. It is the medium through which education either travels or dissolves.

And that means the educator's job is not just to build good programs. It is to tend to the environment in which those programs live. To notice what the informal moments are communicating. To be present in the spaces between the scheduled ones. To understand that every interaction (every hallway conversation, every response to a question, every moment of recognition or its absence) is an education act, whether it was designed to be or not.

That is what it means to be a culture keeper. And it is, I have come to believe, the most important part of the job.

What Culture Actually Is

Culture is one of those words that gets used so often in organizational conversations that it starts to lose its meaning. We talk about building culture, changing culture, protecting culture, and somewhere in all that talking, the actual substance of what culture is and how it works gets lost.

So let me be specific.

Culture is the sum of what people experience when they are part of your department. Not what the mission statement says. Not what the values are called on the poster in the break room. What people actually feel, day after day, in the accumulated texture of how things work here: how mistakes are handled, how questions are received, how recognition is given, how conflict is navigated, how new people are welcomed, how experienced people are treated when they are struggling.

Edgar Schein, one of the foundational researchers on organizational culture, described it as the pattern of shared assumptions that a group has learned: the way we do things around here, operating largely below the level of conscious awareness. Culture is not decided in a meeting. It is built in moments. Thousands of small moments, over time, that establish the unspoken rules of what is safe, what is valued, and what is possible in this place.

What this means for the clinical educator is both empowering and sobering.

It is empowering because it means culture is changeable: not through grand gestures or strategic initiatives alone, but through the consistent, intentional accumulation of small moments that tell a different story than the old one. One recognition that is specific and public. One "What's Broken?" conversation where the feedback is actually acted on. One moment of genuine psychological safety where an RT speaks up and is met with engagement rather than dismissal. These moments accumulate. They become the new pattern. They become the culture.

It is sobering because it means the educator is always building culture, whether intentionally or not. Every impatient response to a question. Every moment of recognition withheld. Every "that's just how it is here" that closes a conversation instead of opening it. These moments accumulate too. And left unexamined, they build a culture that undermines everything the formal education program is trying to create.

The culture keeper's job is to be conscious of both and to choose, consistently and intentionally, the moments that build rather than the ones that erode.

Recognition That Actually Lands

Let me tell you something about recognition that most departments get wrong.

Generic recognition does not work.

A "good job" in passing. An "employee of the month" plaque with a standard citation. A group email thanking "the team" for their hard work during a difficult stretch. These things are not harmful. They are simply insufficient because they do not communicate what recognition is actually for: not reward but witness. The message that someone in authority saw specifically what you did and understood specifically why it mattered.

Recognition that lands is specific. It names the behavior, not just the outcome. It is delivered close to the moment it was earned, not saved for the annual review. And it is public enough to communicate to the whole department what the organization values, not just private enough to make one person feel good.

Here is what it sounds like:

"I want to take a moment to recognize what Marcus did on Tuesday night. He was three hours into a solo shift when he caught a subtle change in a patient's waveform that the monitor hadn't alarmed on yet. He escalated appropriately, stayed calm, and communicated clearly, and that patient got the intervention they needed before the situation became a crisis. That is clinical reasoning. That is exactly what we are building here. Marcus, I see you."

That recognition does several things simultaneously. It tells Marcus that his clinical judgment is visible and valued. It tells every other RT in the room what clinical reasoning looks like in practice better than any competency module could. It reinforces the culture of thinking rather than just doing. And it communicates to the whole department that this is a place where excellence is noticed.

None of that requires a budget. It requires presence (being close enough to the clinical work to see what is happening) and intention (choosing to name it out loud rather than letting it pass unremarked).

The Shout-Out Wall is a practical extension of this principle. A physical or digital space where anyone, not just leadership, can post recognition for a colleague. "Shout out to Priya for staying forty-five minutes after her shift to help a new graduate work through a difficult case." "Shout out to the night team for their teamwork during last week's NICU emergency." Simple. Visible. Democratizing recognition so that it flows laterally through the department, peer to peer, not just vertically from leadership down.

When recognition becomes a department practice rather than a leadership function, something shifts. Staff start noticing each other. The culture of appreciation becomes self-sustaining, not dependent on the educator or the manager to keep it alive, but embedded in the daily habits of the team.

That is a culture keeper's deepest goal: to build practices that outlast their own direct involvement.

The "What's Broken?" Huddle

Here is a question that most departments are afraid to ask their staff:

"What is one thing about our workflow, our culture, or our department that is frustrating you right now?"

Afraid, because asking invites answers. And answers require responses. And responses require action. And action requires the organizational willingness to actually change something based on what staff say, which is harder and more disruptive than simply not asking.

But here is what happens when you don't ask: staff tell each other instead. The frustration that might have become a constructive suggestion in a supported conversation becomes a complaint in the break room. The workflow problem that a staff RT has already solved in their head (because they live inside it every day and they can see exactly what is wrong and exactly what would fix it) stays unsolved because nobody ever created a space where the solution could be offered.

The "What's Broken?" huddle is that space.

It is simple. Once a month, in a brief, structured conversation (a staff meeting, a huddle, a Preceptor Power Hour), you ask the question. Not as a complaint forum. As a problem-solving invitation. "What is one thing we could do differently that would make this department work better for our patients or for our team?"

Then, and this is the part that separates a "What's Broken?" huddle from an empty suggestion box, you fix one thing. Every month. Not every suggestion. One. The most actionable, the most impactful, the one that sends the clearest signal that this conversation is real.

And you name who suggested it.

"Last month, Tanya pointed out that our handoff communication process was creating gaps in treatment continuity for patients transitioning from the ICU to the step-down unit. We made a change to the handoff protocol based on her suggestion. Here is what is different, and here is why it matters."

That sequence (ask, act, attribute) does something that no engagement survey or culture initiative can replicate. It demonstrates, through concrete action, that staff voice has weight here. That the people closest to the work are trusted to identify what needs to change. That this department belongs, in a meaningful sense, to everyone who works in it, not just to the people with offices.

The RT who sees their suggestion implemented, who hears their name attached to an improvement that makes their colleagues' work better and their patients' care safer, does not experience that as a minor workplace perk. They experience it as a professional agency. As the felt sense that what they think, notice, and care about actually matters here.

That feeling is one of the most powerful retention forces available to any department. And it is built one "What's Broken?" conversation at a time.

Psychological Safety: The Foundation of Everything

We have returned to psychological safety many times throughout this book: in the clinical reasoning chapters, in the preceptor development work, in the leadership conversations. I want to address it here, in the context of culture, because it is the foundation on which everything else rests.

Amy Edmondson's research on psychological safety (the belief that one will not be punished or humiliated for speaking up with ideas, questions, concerns, or mistakes) has demonstrated consistently that it is the single strongest predictor of team learning and performance in complex, high-stakes environments. Healthcare teams with high psychological safety catch errors earlier, learn faster, and perform better under pressure than those without it.

In a respiratory therapy department, psychological safety looks like this:

The new graduate who is unsure about a ventilator setting asks their preceptor out loud, in front of a patient, rather than guessing and hoping.

The experienced RT who disagrees with a physician's order brings the concern to the team rather than complying silently and documenting the outcome.

The charge therapist who made a scheduling error acknowledges it directly rather than deflecting or minimizing.

The staff RT who has an idea for improving the department's approach to rapid response preparation brings it to a staff meeting rather than sharing it only in the break room.

None of these behaviors happen in environments where speaking up has historically been costly. They happen where the consistent, demonstrated experience of the team is: *Your voice is welcome here. Your uncertainty is information, not weakness. Your mistakes are learning opportunities, not verdicts.*

Building that environment is the culture keeper's most important long-term work. It cannot be declared into existence. It is built through the consistent modeling of the leader who asks questions rather than performing certainty. Who responds to errors with curiosity before judgment. Who celebrates the RT who admitted uncertainty and sought help at least as publicly as the RT who performed brilliantly under pressure.

And it is protected, fiercely, consistently, whenever something threatens it. The dismissive response to a question. The public criticism of a clinical decision. The eye roll that communicates "You should already know this." These are not small moments. They are cultural messages. And a culture keeper who allows them to pass without addressing them has allowed the foundation to crack.

Building Bridges Beyond the Department: The Clinical Collaboration Summit

There is a gap that exists in respiratory therapy education that nobody talks about loudly enough.

It is the gap between what academic programs teach and what clinical sites expect. Between the skills and frameworks students develop in the classroom and the skills and frameworks their preceptors assume they already have when they arrive for their rotation. Between the curriculum the Director of Clinical Education designed and the orientation the clinical educator built: two systems that are supposed to connect seamlessly but often don't connect at all.

Students feel this gap most acutely. They arrive at their clinical rotation having learned one set of expectations, only to encounter another. Preceptors feel it too, frustrated when students don't know things they assumed would be covered, uncertain about what the academic program has and hasn't addressed. And DCEs feel it from the other side: designing curriculum without always knowing what clinical sites need, sending students into environments they haven't been able to fully prepare them for.

Everyone is working hard. Nobody is working together.

The Clinical Collaboration Summit is my answer to that gap.

Once a year, I bring everyone into the same room. Academic partners: the DCEs from the programs whose students rotate through our department. Clinical preceptors: the Tier Two, Three, and Four preceptors who will actually be working with those students. Department leadership. And myself as the bridge between all of them.

The agenda is simple, and the purpose is singular: alignment.

We discuss what academic programs are teaching and when, so preceptors understand what foundation students are arriving with and can build on it rather than duplicate or contradict it. We discuss what the clinical site expects so DCEs can prepare students more specifically for what they will actually encounter. We discuss the transition from student to orientee: the specific moments when the gap tends to surface and what both sides can do to close it.

And then something happens that I did not fully anticipate the first time I ran it.

The preceptors ask questions.

Not to the DCEs as adversaries or critics, but as partners. "What do your students struggle with most when they arrive? What do you wish we knew about how they've been trained? What would help you prepare them better for what we're going to ask of them?" These are not defensive questions. They are collaborative ones. They are the questions of people who suddenly realize that their clinical site and the academic programs that feed it are part of the same system, and that the system works better when everyone in it is talking to each other.

The DCEs ask questions too. "What do your best orientees have that your struggling ones don't?" "What could we emphasize more in the curriculum that would make a difference?" "What does a student who is truly ready for your department look like?"

By the end of the Summit, something has shifted. The gap that nobody was talking about is now a shared problem with shared ownership. The academic partners and the clinical site are no longer two separate institutions sending and receiving students across an invisible divide. They are collaborators: aligned on expectations, invested in each other's success, connected by the shared commitment to the student standing in the middle of it all.

This Summit is something I plan to hold annually. Not because it is required. Because it works.

And the evidence is in the applications.

When students rotate through a department where the preceptors are prepared for them specifically, where the clinical expectations align with what they learned in school, where the environment feels coherent rather than contradictory, where someone has clearly thought through how to make their transition successful, they notice. They tell their classmates. They come back.

Ninety-five percent of them applied.

That number did not come from a recruitment strategy. It came from a culture, one that extends beyond the department walls into the academic partnerships that shape every student before they ever walk through the door. One that treats the clinical-academic relationship not as a transactional arrangement but as a genuine collaboration in service of the profession's future.

That is what connecting the dots looks like in practice.

And it starts with getting everyone in the same room.

Building Your Own Clinical Collaboration Summit

You do not need a large budget or a formal program to begin. You need the willingness to make the invitation and the commitment to follow through on what you hear.

Who to invite: DCEs from every academic program whose students rotate through your department. Your active preceptors, especially Tier Two and above. Your department supervisor or manager. Yourself as facilitator.

When to hold it: Annually, ideally before the new rotation cycle begins. Give yourself and your academic partners enough lead time to act on what you learn before the next cohort of students arrives.

What to cover:

What students are learning academically and when: a curriculum overview from each DCE.

What the clinical site expects: your orientation structure, preceptor tier system, and developmental philosophy.

Where the gaps are: An honest conversation about what students typically struggle with and why.

What both sides can do differently: Specific, actionable commitments from both the academic program and the clinical site.

How you will stay connected between summits: Email, check-ins, shared documentation.

What to do after: Follow through. Implement what you committed to. Share the outcomes with your academic partners. And hold the Summit again next year, because alignment is not a one-time achievement. It is an ongoing practice.

The Clinical Collaboration Summit is culture keeping at its widest radius. It extends the intentional, development-focused environment you have built inside your department outward, into the academic relationships that determine who walks through your door, how prepared they are, and whether the gap they experience when they arrive builds them up or breaks them down.

Close the gap. Build the bridge. Connect the dots.

That is the culture keeper's work, inside the department and beyond it.

The Proof

I want to close this chapter with something concrete. Not a framework, a tool, or a reflection prompt, though those follow. A result.

After implementing the practices described in this book (the tiered preceptor system, the Preceptor Power Hours, the badges, the two-way daily evaluations, the Level Up Week, the clinical reasoning culture, the recognition practices, the career conversations), something measurable happened in my department.

The number of students choosing us for their clinical rotations tripled. And then something even more significant happened: ninety-five percent of them applied for positions after graduation.

Not because we advertised differently. Not because our compensation package changed. Because students who rotated through our department experienced something they had not experienced anywhere else. And when I asked them (as I always do, because the feedback loop never closes), they told me, in different words and consistent themes, the same thing:

The preceptors actually wanted to teach.

The environment was different.

Those two sentences are the summary of this entire book.

Preceptors who want to teach are not born. They are developed: through intentional preparation, Preceptor Power Hours, and a clear expectation that teaching is a professional skill worthy of the same investment we bring to clinical skill. Through being given a badge that says their role matters and a clinical ladder that says their growth does too.

An environment that feels different is not accidental. It is built: through recognition that is specific and public, conversations that ask what is broken and actually fix it, daily modeling of psychological safety by every leader at every level. Through an educator who understands that her job happens in the hallways as much as in the classrooms, in the informal moments as much as the formal ones, in the small accumulated choices that, over time, become the culture of a department.

Students came. They experienced something real. They applied.

That is retention before it begins. That is the culture keeper's work: building an environment so compelling, so genuinely invested in the development of its people, that the people choose it. Not because they have no other options.

Because this place is worth choosing.

Chapter Summary

- The educator's role extends far beyond orientation logistics. What happens in the informal moments (the hallways, the break rooms, the five-minute conversations) shapes department culture as powerfully as any formal education program.

- Culture is built in small moments. Specific recognition. Honest conversations. Psychological safety modeled consistently. The accumulation of these moments becomes the pattern (the way things are done here) that either attracts and retains people or quietly drives them away.
- Recognition that lands is specific, timely, and public. It names the behavior, not just the outcome, and communicates to the whole department what is valued here.
- The "What's Broken?" huddle (ask, act, attribute) transforms staff frustration into department ownership. One thing fixed every month, with the suggester's name attached, builds the felt sense that this department belongs to everyone in it.
- Psychological safety is the foundation of everything. It cannot be declared; it must be consistently modeled and fiercely protected.
- The Clinical Collaboration Summit (an annual gathering of academic partners, clinical preceptors, and department leadership) closes the gap between what academic programs teach and what clinical sites expect. Alignment between the two creates a coherent, supported student experience that drives applications and retention before the hire even happens.

- The proof: when preceptors want to teach and the environment feels different, students notice. They apply. Retention begins before the hire, in the clinical rotation experience of a student who feels something they haven't anywhere else.

Reflection Prompts

1. Think about the informal moments in your department (the hallways, the break rooms, the brief interactions between scheduled education events). What are those moments communicating about the culture you are building?
2. When was the last time you gave recognition that was specific enough to name the exact behavior and explain exactly why it mattered? What stopped you from doing it more consistently?
3. Does your department have a regular, structured space where staff can name what is broken and where they see evidence that what they say is acted upon? If not, what would it take to create one?
4. Think about the academic programs whose students rotate through your department. When was the last time you sat in the same room with their DCEs and your preceptors to align expectations? What would change if you did?

Coming Up in Chapter Twelve

We have built the culture keeper's toolkit (recognition, the "What's Broken?" huddle, and the psychological safety that makes everything else possible). In Chapter

Twelve, we turn to one of the most honest and difficult conversations in the STAY pillar: what to do when the culture is broken, when the environment you are trying to build is working against forces larger than any single educator can easily move and how to start somewhere anyway.

"Preceptors who want to teach are not born. They are developed. An environment that feels different is not accidental. It is built."

12

THE EDUCATOR'S SURVIVAL GUIDE

You Cannot Pour from an Empty Cup, But Nobody Asks If Yours Is Full

> *"You have to keep breaking your heart until it opens."*
> *– Rumi*

Nobody Asked

I want to ask you something I suspect nobody has asked you recently.

Are you okay?

Not "are you managing?" Not "are you keeping up?" Not "is everything on track with the orientation schedule?" Are you, the person behind the educator role, the human being who shows up every day to pour into everyone else, actually okay?

I ask because I know what it is like to be the person everyone comes to. The one who holds the new RT who is overwhelmed, the preceptor who is struggling, the staff member who needs to be heard, the manager who needs a problem solved, and the student who is terrified, all in the same week, sometimes in the same day. I know what it is like to be so focused on filling everyone else's cup that the question of whether your own is empty never quite makes it to the top of the priority list.

And I know that rarely, almost never, in my experience, does anyone stop and ask the educator if she is okay.

Not because the people around you don't care. But because you are so consistently capable, so reliably present, so apparently fine that the question doesn't seem necessary. You have made competence look effortless. And, from the outside, effortless does not look like it needs tending.

But it does. You do.

This chapter is for you: the educator, the preceptor developer, the culture keeper, the person who has been building everything described in this book while simultaneously figuring out how to sustain yourself through the building. It is the chapter that asks not what you owe your department but what you owe yourself. And it makes the argument, plainly and without apology, that your development is not a luxury. It is a professional responsibility. Because the educator who stops growing stops being able to develop others. And the educator who stops being cared for eventually stops being able to care.

The Conference Moment

I want to tell you about a conference.

I attended, as I try to do, because professional gatherings are one of the few places where the specific loneliness of the clinical educator role briefly dissolves. There were two tracks. Academic educators. Leadership.

Both were valuable. Both offered connection, networking, and the particular relief of being in a room with people who understand, at least partially, what this work involves.

But I sat in those sessions and felt something I had felt before: a specific kind of professional hunger that neither track was quite feeding. I was not purely an academic educator. I was not purely in a leadership role. I was something in between and beyond both: a hospital-based clinical educator whose role touched every aspect of department development and whose specific developmental needs did not map cleanly onto either of the available options.

So I said something. In the room, out loud, to people I had just met.

"This is wonderful for networking. But who do I learn from? Who mentors me?"

The question landed in the silence that follows when someone names something everyone has been feeling but nobody has said. Heads nodded. The conversation that followed was one of the most honest and energizing professional exchanges I had experienced in years.

Nobody had an answer. Not because the answer didn't exist, but because the infrastructure for developing hospital-based RT educators the way we develop the RTs they educate simply does not yet exist at scale. There is no formal track. No established mentorship pipeline. No "here is how you become better at this specific role" that you can follow the way a new graduate follows an orientation plan.

What I did with that absence is, I think, the most important thing I have ever done for my professional development.

I became the answer for others and built my own development from everything and everyone around me.

Building Yourself When No One Builds You

Here is what I did. Not as a prescription (every educator's path will look different), but as a testimony to what is possible when you refuse to wait for someone else to design your development.

I looked at the people in my life who were excellent at adjacent things and I asked them to teach me.

My husband is an assistant principal. He understands instructional design, classroom management, adult learning, and the particular challenge of developing people within institutions that do not always support what development requires. I talked to him (really talked, the way you talk to someone who will be honest with you) about what he had learned and what he wished someone had told him earlier. I applied it.

My best friend is a department chair of a respiratory therapy program. She understands the academic side of RT education from the inside out: the curriculum design, the student development frameworks, the gap between classroom and clinical that both of us were trying to close from different directions. We talked. We challenged each other. We became, informally and powerfully, each other's most relevant professional mentors.

Close friends who had grown, who had navigated their own professional development in their own fields with wisdom and humility, shared what they wished they had known. Not respiratory therapy wisdom specifically. Human wisdom. Leadership wisdom. The kind that transfers across disciplines because it is grounded in what it means to develop people, build cultures, and sustain yourself through the long work of both.

And I prayed. I want to say that plainly, without qualification, because it is true and because it is part of my story and because the educator who is reading this and finding sustenance in faith deserves to see that named rather than omitted. Prayer was part of how I refilled. Part of how I found direction when the path was unclear. Part of how I kept going when the cup felt empty and nobody had noticed.

And then I read.

I read voraciously, across disciplines, pulling from every source that could teach me something about the work I was doing:

How to Teach Healthcare Professionals, because someone had thought carefully about the specific challenges of clinical education and I needed to learn from them.

Start With Why by Simon Sinek, because understanding purpose is the foundation of every culture-building conversation I would ever have.

The Leadership Challenge by Kouzes and Posner, because leadership is a learnable practice, and I needed its framework.

Teach Like a Champion by Doug Lemov, because the specific craft of teaching (the moves, the habits, the intentional practices) had been studied and documented, and I wanted to know what had been learned.

Emotional Intelligence by Daniel Goleman, because the work of developing people is fundamentally relational, and I needed to understand what that required of me emotionally.

The 7 Habits of Highly Effective People by Stephen Covey, because effectiveness is built on principles, and I needed mine to be clear.

And more. Always more. The educator who stops reading stops having new things to offer. And I was not willing to stop.

Alongside the reading, I pursued credentials. Not because letters after my name were the point, but because learning is the point, and structured learning programs are one of the most efficient ways to build expertise systematically. After twenty years away from formal education, I returned to school and completed my Bachelor of Science. Then my ACCS. Then my NPS. Then my MBA. Then my Lean Practitioner certification. All within a two-year span that my husband will tell you was ambitious, that my sons will tell you was intense, and that I will tell you was the most intellectually alive I had felt in years.

I was not waiting for someone to develop me. I was developing myself from every available source across every discipline that had something to teach me, at a pace that matched the urgency I felt about the work I was trying to do.

That pace is not one I recommend for everyone. It is the pace that was right for me, in that season, driven by that particular hunger. What I do recommend, for every educator reading this, is the underlying commitment. The decision that your development is your responsibility. That the absence of a formal track is not an excuse to stop growing. That the resources exist in the people around you, in the books on the shelf, in the conferences where you speak up and ask the uncomfortable question, if you are willing to look for them and use them.

Finding Your People

The loneliness of the clinical educator role is real.

There is often only one of you in a department. You sit at the intersection of clinical practice and education, of staff development and leadership, of orientation logistics and culture building, and that intersection is a genuinely unusual place to occupy. Most of your colleagues are either clinicians or administrators. Very few understand the specific texture of what you do or the specific challenges it produces.

This is why finding your people, the community of educators who inhabit the same intersection, matters as much as any skill or credential you can develop.

The AARC is the obvious starting point. The annual congress, the summer forum, the state affiliate meetings: these are the spaces where RT educators gather, where the national conversation about workforce development and clinical education happens, where you can find the peers, mentors, and collaborators that your department cannot provide.

But finding your people also means being willing to build community where it doesn't yet exist. To speak up at the conference and ask the uncomfortable question. To connect on LinkedIn with the educator in another state who is doing similar work. To reach out to the DCE at the academic program whose students you work with and say, not just in the context of the Clinical Collaboration Summit but as a genuine professional relationship, "I think we can learn from each other."

I built a presence on LinkedIn as the Friendly Educator, not as a marketing strategy but as a professional identity. A way of saying, publicly and consistently: this is who I am, this is what I care about, this is the work I am doing and why it matters. That presence brought people to me: other educators, clinicians, leaders, and students who were doing similar work and asking similar questions, and who, over time, became a genuine professional community.

Your community may look different. Build it anyway. Because the educator who is trying to do this work alone (without peers who understand it, without mentors who can challenge her, without the particular sustenance of knowing that someone else gets it) is carrying a weight that no single person should carry indefinitely.

Advocating for Your Role

Here is something I want to say directly to every hospital-based clinical educator reading this book:

Your role is not fully understood by most of the institutions that employ you. And that misunderstanding has consequences for your resources, your recognition, your ability to do the work that this book describes.

Most hospitals understand the clinical educator as an orientation coordinator. Someone who manages onboarding paperwork, schedules competency verifications, and ensures that new hires are cleared for independent practice in the required timeframe. This is a transactional understanding of a transformational role, and it produces transactional support. Limited protected time. Minimal professional development budget. Little organizational investment in the educator's own growth.

The educator who accepts that understanding without challenge has, inadvertently, agreed to a ceiling on what she can accomplish.

Advocating for your role means making the case, specifically and with data, to the people who control resources, for what your role actually is and what it requires to do well. It means bringing the retention data and saying: "Here is the cost of turnover. Here is how intentional development reduces it. Here is what I need to build the program that produces those outcomes." It means documenting the results (the 95% application rate, the Level Up Week survey feedback, the preceptor satisfaction data) and presenting them as evidence of return on investment.

It means asking for the protected time, the conference attendance, the certification support, the dedicated space, not apologetically, but as a professional making the case for what the work requires.

No one will advocate for the educator's role if the educator does not. And the work described in this book (the tiered preceptor system, the Power Hours, the Clinical Reasoning Passport, the Level Up Week, the Clinical Collaboration Summit) cannot be built in the margins of a role that has been defined too narrowly to contain it.

Define it yourself. Build the case. Ask for what you need. And keep asking until the institution understands what it has in you.

Staying Current Without Burning Out

The field moves. New evidence. New equipment. New credentialing requirements. New generations of learners with new learning styles and new expectations. The educator who was current three years ago and has not been investing in her own learning since is already behind, not through negligence, but through the relentless forward motion of a field that does not pause for the people trying to keep up with it.

Staying current without burning out requires a different relationship with professional development than most educators have been taught to have.

It is not about consuming everything. It is about consuming strategically: identifying the areas most relevant to your current work and your developing practice, and going deep there rather than wide everywhere. One journal. One conference. One book per quarter. One new practice implemented and evaluated before the next one is adopted.

It is about building learning into the rhythm of the work rather than stacking it on top. The Preceptor Power Hour where you facilitate a discussion on a topic you are also learning about. The Level Up Week station you host on content you spent two weeks reviewing. The LinkedIn post you write about a clinical education concept that forces you to articulate what you think, because writing is one of the most effective forms of learning available to anyone at any stage of their career.

And it is about permitting yourself to not know everything. The educator who projects omniscience (who presents herself as the authority on all things rather than the facilitator of collective learning) has set herself an unsustainable standard and, not incidentally, has modeled for her department that uncertainty is something to be hidden rather than navigated.

The educator who says, "I've been reading about this, and here's what I'm learning. What do you think?" is not displaying weakness. She is modeling exactly the culture of intellectual curiosity and continuous growth that she is trying to instill in everyone around her.

Stay curious. Stay humble. Stay current, not perfectly, not exhaustively, but consistently and intentionally. And give yourself the same grace you give your new graduates when they are learning something hard.

You are always learning something hard. That is what this work requires. And it is, in its own demanding way, one of the greatest privileges of the role.

What You Need: A Direct Inventory

I want to close this chapter with something practical. Not a framework. A list. A direct, honest inventory of what the clinical educator needs to sustain herself and keep growing. Not what the institution provides. What you need, and what you have the right to ask for.

Time. Protected, dedicated time for your own professional development. Not the margins of the day. Actual scheduled time that is understood by your department as an investment in the educator who is building everything else.

Community. At least one peer who understands this specific role (another hospital-based educator, a DCE, a mentor in an adjacent field) with whom you can be honest about the hard parts without performing capability you don't always feel.

Resources. Conference attendance. Certification support. Access to the literature and the professional organizations that are advancing the field. These are not perks. They are tools.

Recognition. The acknowledgment, from your institution, your colleagues, and yourself, that what you do is extraordinary. That the culture you build, the preceptors you develop, the new RTs whose trajectories you shape: this is significant work. It deserves to be named as such.

Rest. Real rest. The kind that is not guilty, provisional, or interrupted by the mental list of everything that still needs doing. The educator who cannot rest cannot sustain. And the educator who cannot sustain cannot build the things this book describes.

Faith. In whatever form that takes for you. The sustaining belief that this work matters. That the individual you invested in today will invest in someone else tomorrow. That the profession is better because you showed up, and will be better still because you keep showing up.

You give all of these things to the people you develop. You deserve them too.

Ask for them. Receive them. And keep going.

Chapter Summary

- Nobody asks the educator if she is okay. This chapter does, and makes the case that the educator's wellbeing, growth, and sustainability are not personal concerns but professional responsibilities.
- When no formal development track exists for your specific role, you build your own, from the people around you, the books on your shelf, the

conferences where you ask the uncomfortable question, and the credentials that deepen your expertise.

- Finding your people, a community of educators who understand the specific intersection you occupy, is as important as any skill or credential you can develop. Build it actively, not passively.
- Advocating for your role means making the case with data, with results, with professional clarity, for what the role actually requires. Nobody else will define it if you don't.
- Staying current without burning out requires strategic depth over exhaustive breadth: learning intentionally, building it into the rhythm of the work, and modeling the intellectual humility you want to see in your department.
- What you need: time, community, resources, recognition, rest, and faith. You give all of these to the people you develop. You deserve them too.

Reflection Prompts

1. When was the last time someone asked if you were okay, really okay? And when was the last time you asked yourself honestly?
2. Who are your people, the community that understands this specific role? If you don't have them yet, where would you start building?

3. What does your current professional development look like? Is it strategic and sustainable, or is it either exhausting or absent?

4. What do you need from your institution that you have not yet asked for? What is stopping you from asking?

5. What would you tell a new clinical educator, someone stepping into this role for the first time, about how to survive and thrive in it? That answer is also a letter to yourself.

Coming Up in Chapter Thirteen

We have cared for the educator. In Chapter Thirteen, we zoom out to the practical architecture of sustained development: the Post-Orientation Development Plan. Because orientation ends. Learning should not. And the thirty-sixty-ninety-day framework that bridges the gap between competency and capability is the structure that makes everything this book has described sustainable beyond the first ninety days.

*"Nobody asked the educator if she was okay.
This chapter does. Because you cannot pour from
an empty cup, and you have been pouring for a long time."*

13

THE POST-ORIENTATION DEVELOPMENT PLAN

Orientation Ends. Learning Should Not.

"The end of orientation is not the finish line.
It is the starting line."

Dropped Off in the Middle of Nowhere

She came to me after orientation ended.

Not with a clinical question. Not with a competency concern. With something harder to name and, in some ways, harder to address: a feeling.

She told me that when orientation ended, it felt like she had been dropped off in the middle of nowhere.

She had done everything right. She had completed the competencies, passed the evaluations, built relationships with her preceptors, and demonstrated the clinical skills required to practice independently. By every formal measure, she was ready. The paperwork said so. The signatures said so.

But the day she walked onto the floor without a preceptor beside her, the first shift of true independence, the moment that every new RT has been working toward and dreading simultaneously, something happened that no orientation plan had prepared her for.

The silence. Not literal silence: the floor was busy, the patients needed care, the work continued exactly as it had during orientation. But the silence of no longer having a structured relationship that held her. No preceptor whose presence communicated: you are not alone in this. No formal check-in scheduled for the end of the shift. No Clinical Reasoning Passport entry to write. No Preceptor Power Hour to look forward to. Just her, and the patients, and the sudden awareness that the scaffolding had been removed and she was now standing entirely on her own.

She was not struggling clinically. She was struggling with the transition, with the specific vulnerability of moving from supported learner to independent practitioner, without any formal acknowledgment that the transition itself is hard, that the silence that follows orientation is real, and that needing support after orientation ends is not a sign of inadequacy but a completely normal human response to a genuinely significant professional threshold.

She told me what she needed. And I listened.

And then I built the mentoring program.

That is what this chapter is about: the system that catches new RTs in the silence after orientation. The structured, sustained, human connection that says: *Orientation may have ended, but your development hasn't. And neither has our investment in you.*

The Cliff Nobody Plans For

We have discussed throughout this book the 12-Month Cliff, the predictable spike in RT turnover that occurs between twelve and eighteen months of employment. We have talked about its causes: the plateau that follows the initial learning curve, the absence of visible growth pathways, the quiet disengagement of someone who has become competent enough to know they could find something better.

But there is an earlier cliff that receives even less attention.

It happens at the end of orientation.

The day the formal structure ends, the new RT steps into a professional landscape that looks almost identical to the one they have been practicing in (same floor, same patients, same colleagues, same equipment) but feels fundamentally different. The difference is invisible from the outside and unmistakable from within. The structured support is gone. The formal relationship that held the learning is over. The new RT is, for the first time, professionally alone in a way they have not been since their very first day.

Most departments have not planned for this moment. They have planned for orientation. They have designed the competency verification, the preceptor relationship, and the skills progression. And then orientation ends, the new RT is cleared for independent practice, and the developmental conversation effectively stops until the annual performance review, or until something goes wrong.

The gap between orientation ending and the first formal follow-up is, in many departments, months long. And in those months (in the early weeks of independent practice when the new RT is most vulnerable, most uncertain, and most likely to encounter clinical situations that exceed their current capability), they are navigating alone.

The Post-Orientation Development Plan closes that gap. Not by extending orientation indefinitely: that would defeat the purpose of independent practice. But by replacing the formal structure of orientation with a different kind of structure: lighter, more flexible, built for a practitioner rather than a learner, but present enough to ensure that the silence after orientation is never abandonment.

The Architecture: Five Touchpoints That Change Everything

The post-orientation support system I have built in my department has five components that work together to sustain the new RT through the most vulnerable stretch of their early career. Each one serves a distinct purpose. Together they form a net, not one that prevents the new RT from standing on their own, but one that ensures they never have to fall very far alone.

The 30-Day Check-In: Building the Habit of Reflection

Thirty days after orientation ends, the new RT sits down with me for a structured conversation. Not a performance review. Not a competency evaluation. A developmental check-in, focused entirely on how the transition to independent practice is going and what the new RT needs to continue growing.

The questions are specific and unhurried:

"What has been the hardest part of working independently? What surprised you?"

"Tell me about a clinical situation in the last thirty days that pushed you. What did you do, and what did you learn?"

"What questions are you carrying that you haven't been able to answer yet?"

"What do you need from me, from your preceptor, or from the department right now that you're not currently getting?"

That last question is the most important. And the answer, whatever it is, becomes the agenda for the next thirty days.

The 30-day check-in also serves a monitoring function that I want to name directly. The new RT who is struggling clinically in the first thirty days of independent practice is not always visible from the outside. They are often performing adequately while quietly carrying uncertainty that has not yet surfaced. The structured check-in creates a space where that uncertainty can emerge, where the RT can say "I'm not sure I handled that situation correctly" or "I've been second-guessing myself more than I expected" without fear of formal consequence. And what surfaces in that space can be addressed before it becomes a patient safety concern or a retention crisis.

The 60-Day Check-In: Expanding Scope and Voice

By sixty days, the new RT has found some footing. The floor is familiar. The patients are less uniformly terrifying. The clinical tasks that required conscious effort are beginning to feel more automatic.

This is the moment (not later, not at the annual review) to begin expanding the conversation from survival to growth.

The 60-day check-in asks different questions from the 30-day one:

"You've been independent for sixty days. What kind of clinician are you becoming? Describe yourself, not your skills, but your thinking."

"What clinical area or patient population do you want to understand more deeply? What would it take to get there?"

"Where have you led this month, even informally, even without a title? Did you notice it?"

"What's one thing you want to do differently in the next thirty days?"

The shift in these questions, from "how are you surviving" to "how are you growing," communicates something important to the new RT. It says: *We are not just watching to make sure you don't fall. We are invested in where you go.* That message, delivered at sixty days when the initial survival anxiety is beginning to ease, is one of the most powerful retention interventions available. It arrives at exactly the moment when the new RT is starting to look up from the immediate demands of the work and ask the bigger question: is this where I want to be?

The answer they receive to that question in the sixty-day check-in shapes how they answer the bigger one.

The 90-Day Milestone: Owning the Path Forward

The ninety-day check-in is a milestone, not just a meeting. It marks the formal transition from new RT to established staff member, and it deserves to be treated with the intentionality that milestone implies.

I do three things at the ninety-day check-in that I do not do at the thirty- or sixty-day ones.

I celebrate. Specifically, publicly if appropriate, with genuine acknowledgment of what the RT has accomplished: not just the competencies they cleared but the growth they demonstrated, the moments that revealed their clinical reasoning developing, the ways they showed up for patients and colleagues that the formal record does not capture.

I close the Clinical Reasoning Passport. Not by taking it away (it belongs to the RT), but by reviewing it together, one last time, as a developmental record. We read early entries alongside recent ones. We name the growth out loud. And then I ask the RT to write one final entry: "What kind of clinician am I becoming?" That entry, written at ninety days, is one of the most powerful documents in the passport, because it captures, in the RT's own words, the professional identity that has been forming over three months of guided reflection.

And I introduce the next phase. The clinical ladder. The specialty certification pathway. The leadership ladder and where the RT might begin climbing it. The mentorship pair that will continue beyond this check-in. The 6-month and 1-year conversations already on the calendar.

Because the ninety-day check-in is not the end. It is the transition to a different kind of beginning.

The Manager's Check-Ins: Senior Leadership in the Conversation

Here is the element of our post-orientation system that I believe makes the most significant difference in how new RTs experience their early careers, and that most departments have not thought to include.

Our department manager sits down with every new RT at thirty, sixty, and ninety days as well.

Not instead of my check-ins. In addition to them. Separately scheduled, with her own questions and her own relational presence, because the message that a department manager's direct, unhurried attention sends to a new RT is qualitatively different from the message that even the most invested educator can send.

It says: *You matter to this organization at the highest level of this department. Not just to the person whose job it is to develop you. To the person who leads this team.*

That message, delivered in the intimate context of a one-on-one conversation rather than in a group meeting or a department-wide communication, changes how the new RT understands their place in the department. They are not invisible to leadership. They are known. They are valued. The organization has invested enough in their success to ask the person who runs the department to sit down and ask how they are doing.

The manager's check-ins also foster something that no educator-RT relationship alone can fully build: direct communication between the new RT and senior leadership. The RT who has spoken honestly with the department manager at thirty, sixty, and ninety days has a relationship with that leader that changes how they experience the department. They are not strangers who interact only in formal performance contexts. They are people who have had real conversations (about the RT's experience, their needs, their goals, their concerns) and who share a relational foundation that makes every future interaction easier and more honest.

This is culture building at the leadership level. And it is one of the most powerful things a department manager can do with thirty minutes, three times, in the first ninety days of a new RT's career.

The 6-Month and 1-Year Check-Ins: Bridging the 12-Month Cliff

The 12-Month Cliff, as we established in Chapter One, is predictable. And predictable problems deserve proactive solutions.

The 6-month check-in is that solution.

At six months, the new RT is past the acute vulnerability of the early weeks but approaching the territory where disengagement and questioning begin. The excitement of the new role has settled into the reality of the daily work. The initial mentorship intensity has naturally relaxed. The RT is competent, reliably, visibly competent, and for the first time, that competence is not producing the learning energy it did when everything was new.

This is the moment to intervene. Not because something is wrong, but because something is about to become possible if we create the conditions for it.

The 6-month check-in asks:

"You've been here six months. What is still energizing you, and what has started to feel routine?"

"What do you want to learn or do in the next six months that you haven't done yet?"

"Who in this department inspires you professionally? Have you told them?"

"What would make the next six months more meaningful than the last six?"

These questions do not assume a problem. They assume potential and communicate that assumption to the RT, which is itself a form of investment.

The 1-year check-in is both a celebration and a forward-looking conversation. It marks something genuinely significant: a full year of independent practice, survived, navigated, and grown through. It deserves acknowledgment. And it deserves the question that

Chapter Nine identified as the most powerful in the developmental conversation:

"Where do you want to go?"

At one year, with twelve months of real clinical experience behind them and the full context of the department around them, the new RT's answer to that question is specific enough to act on. And acting on it (with a clinical ladder pathway, a certification conversation, a mentorship pairing, a leadership opportunity) is how the 12-Month Cliff becomes a 12-Month Launch.

The Mentoring Program: The Human Infrastructure

Underneath all five of these touchpoints is a human relationship that makes them possible: the mentorship pair.

When that new RT told me she felt dropped off in the middle of nowhere, she was not asking for more check-in meetings. She was asking for a person. Someone who would stay connected to her development not because a schedule required it, but because a relationship sustained it.

The mentoring program pairs every new RT, at the end of orientation, with a mentor, typically a Tier Three or Four preceptor who is not their orientation preceptor, deliberately chosen to create a new relational channel rather than an extension of the existing one. The mentor's role is not clinical supervision. It is developmental companionship. Monthly conversations. A consistent, trusted presence. The person the new RT can call when something happens at 2 a.m. that they are still thinking about at 2 p.m. the next day.

The mentoring relationship is sustained through the first year of independent practice, overlapping with the formal check-ins, complementing manager conversations, and extending the clinical reasoning culture into informal spaces where it often matters most.

And it communicates, more powerfully than any formal structure can, the thing the new RT who felt dropped off in the middle of nowhere most needed to hear:

You are not alone. Not during orientation. Not after it. Not ever, as long as you are part of this department.

What the Plan Looks Like: A Complete Timeline

Here is the full post-orientation development timeline in one place, for every educator who wants to implement it, adapt it, and make it their own.

End of Orientation – Day One of Independence

- Clinical Reasoning Passport remains active
- Mentorship pair officially introduced and first meeting scheduled
- 30-day check-ins with educator AND manager calendared
- New RT receives explicit message: "Orientation ended. Your development didn't."

30 Days Post-Orientation

- Educator check-in: survival, transition, immediate needs
- Manager check-in: relationship building, organizational belonging
- Passport review: What is the new RT writing? What does it reveal?
- Mentorship pair: first formal meeting

60 Days Post-Orientation

- Educator check-in: growth, scope expansion, leadership awareness
- Manager check-in: goals, engagement, early career trajectory
- Passport review: Is reasoning deepening or still task-focused?
- Clinical ladder introduction: Where could this RT go from here?

90 Days Post-Orientation

- Educator check-in: milestone celebration, passport closure, next phase introduction
- Manager check-in: formal recognition, forward-looking conversation
- Specialty certification and leadership pathway conversation begins

6 Months

- 6-month and 1-year check-ins calendared
- Educator check-in: energy, routine, next six months
- Proactive retention conversation: What would make this more meaningful?
- Mentorship pair continues: evolving from survival support to growth partnership

1 Year

- Educator check-in: celebration, reflection, "Where do you want to go?"
- Manager check-in: formal recognition of first-year milestone
- Clinical ladder review: Where is the RT now, and what is the next step?

The 12-Month Cliff becomes the 12-Month Launch.

Chapter Summary

- The silence after orientation ends is real and unplanned for in most departments. A new RT who felt "dropped off in the middle of nowhere" taught us that the transition to independence is its own developmental threshold, requiring its own support structure.

- The Post-Orientation Development Plan has five components: the 30-day check-in, the 60-day check-in, the 90-day milestone, the manager's parallel check-ins, and the 6-month and 1-year conversations that bridge the 12-Month Cliff.
- Manager involvement at 30, 60, and 90 days sends the new RT a message that no educator alone can send: you matter to this organization at the highest level of this department.
- The mentoring program provides the human infrastructure beneath all of the formal touchpoints: a consistent, trusted relationship that says you are not alone, long after orientation ends.
- The 6-month and 1-year check-ins are proactive retention interventions that address the 12-Month Cliff before it becomes a departure. They communicate that the department's investment in the new RT's development does not expire after ninety days.

Reflection Prompts

1. What happens in your department the day after orientation ends? What does the new RT experience, and what does that experience communicate about the department's investment in their development?
2. Is your department manager involved in new RT development beyond formal performance reviews? What would change if they were?

3. How long is the gap, in your department, between orientation ending and the first formal follow-up? What happens to new RTs in that gap?

4. Think about the RT who felt dropped off in the middle of nowhere. Is there one in your department right now, someone in the early weeks of independence who is quietly navigating the silence? What would it take to reach them this week?

Coming Up in Chapter Fourteen

We have built the complete development system, from orientation through the first year and beyond. In Chapter Fourteen, the final chapter before our closing letter, we zoom out to the biggest picture: what this all means for the future of the respiratory therapy profession. Because the work of developing RTs who think, lead, and stay is not just a department strategy. It is a professional legacy.

"Orientation ended. Your development didn't.
And neither did our investment in you."

14

THE REAL MEASURE

A Call to Action for the Respiratory Therapy Profession

"The purpose of life is not to be happy. It is to be useful, to be honorable, to be compassionate,
to have it make some difference that you have lived and lived well."
– Ralph Waldo Emerson

What We Have Built

We have covered a great deal of ground in this book.

We have named the problem: the gap between orientation and education, the preceptor who was never taught to teach, the good RT who left because nobody showed them a path forward. We have built the solution: the clinical reasoning tools, the tiered preceptor system, the Preceptor Power Hours, the Clinical Reasoning Passport, the Level Up Week, the Clinical Collaboration Summit, the post-orientation development plan, the culture of recognition, psychological safety, and belonging that makes all of it sustainable.

We have talked about new graduates and experienced staff, about preceptors and managers, about academic partners and clinical sites. We have talked about the educator's own survival and the profession's collective future. We have told honest stories, cited real research, offered reproducible tools, and asked the uncomfortable questions that most departments have been avoiding.

And now we have arrived at the place every book arrives at eventually: the last chapter before the last page. The moment where the author stops describing and starts challenging.

So here is my challenge.

Not a gentle suggestion. Not a series of action items to consider when time permits. A challenge, direct, urgent, and grounded in twenty years of watching this profession underinvest in its own people while wondering why it can't keep them.

The Profession We Have, and the One We Could Build

Respiratory therapy is one of the most clinically sophisticated, intellectually demanding, and emotionally complex specialties in all of healthcare. We manage the most critical airways, the most fragile lungs, the most vulnerable patients at the most vulnerable moments of their lives. We work in ICUs and NICUs, emergency departments, long-term care facilities, and anywhere else where breathing becomes a crisis. We are, in the truest sense, the specialists of survival.

And we have been treating our own workforce development like an afterthought.

Not maliciously. Not negligently. But consistently, as an institution, as a profession, as a collection of departments that have been so focused on the clinical demands of the work that the human infrastructure required to sustain it has been underfunded, underdesigned, and undervalued for decades.

The result is visible in the data. Turnover rates that exceed what any department can sustainably absorb. New graduates who leave within two years, not because the work isn't meaningful but because nobody made the meaning visible. Experienced clinicians who plateau quietly and depart without fanfare. Preceptors who were assigned a teaching role without being taught to teach. Educators who are building everything described in this book with inadequate time, inadequate resources, and inadequate recognition.

This is not inevitable. It is a choice. And choices can be changed.

The respiratory therapy profession has the clinical knowledge, the professional standards, the national infrastructure, and, in the educators, preceptors, and leaders reading this book, the human talent to build something genuinely different. A profession that develops its people with the same rigor and intention it brings to its clinical practice. A profession where every new RT is given not just a competency checklist but a development plan. Where every preceptor is not just assigned but prepared. Where every experienced clinician is not left to plateau but shown a path forward. Where every educator is not left to build alone but supported, resourced, and recognized for the transformational work they do.

That profession is possible. It is not yet fully built. And building it is the work of every person reading this book.

A Challenge to Educators

If you are a clinical educator, hospital-based, academic, or somewhere in between, this challenge is for you first.

Stop waiting for the system to support you before you begin.

I know the resources are limited. I know the protected time is insufficient. I know the administration does not always understand what you do or why it requires the investment you are asking for. I know because I have lived all of those constraints and built everything in this book within them.

The system will not be fixed before you start. It will be fixed, in part, because you started, because you built results that made the case, documented outcomes that justified the investment, and refused to accept that the absence of perfect conditions was a reason to wait.

Start with one Preceptor Power Hour. One Clinical Reasoning Passport. One "What's Broken?" huddle. One career conversation with an RT who has never been asked where they want to go. One Clinical Collaboration Summit invitation sent to one academic partner.

Start small. Start Monday. And then document what happens, because the results you generate are the argument for everything else you need.

And while you are building, advocate. Loudly, professionally, persistently, for the time, the resources, the recognition, and the organizational support that this role requires. You are not asking for a favor. You are making the business case for the single most cost-effective retention and development investment your department can make.

Make the case. Keep making it. And know that every educator who reads this book and builds something in their department is making the case alongside you, adding to the collective evidence that this work matters and this profession deserves to invest in it.

A Challenge to Department Leaders and Managers

If you are a department leader, a supervisor, a manager, or a director, this challenge is for you.

Get in the room. Not the meeting room. The development room. The Preceptor Power Hour. The 30-day check-in with the new RT who is navigating their first weeks of independence. The Level Up Week station where your most experienced staff are being challenged to explain their clinical reasoning out loud. The Clinical Collaboration Summit where your preceptors are building relationships with the academic partners who send you students.

Get in those rooms. Regularly. Visibly. With genuine presence rather than obligatory attendance.

Because your presence in those rooms sends a message that nothing else can send. It says: *This department's leadership believes that development matters. That preceptors matter. That new RTs matter. That the culture we are building together is worth the time of the people who run this department.*

That message, communicated through consistent, visible presence, changes the energy of every room you walk into. It elevates the Preceptor Power Hour from an educator's initiative to a departmental priority. It tells every preceptor that their development is seen at the highest level. It tells every new RT that they are known, not just managed.

And then act on what you see and hear in those rooms. When an RT brings an idea to the "What's Broken?" huddle, implement it. When a preceptor identifies a gap in their development, address it. When the educator asks for protected time or conference attendance or certification support, say yes, not as a perk but as an investment in the person who is building everything your department needs to thrive.

The leaders who do these things do not just build better departments. They build departments that become known in academic programs, in professional networks, among students who rotate through and apply afterward, as places worth choosing. Places that invest in their people. Places where the preceptors actually want to teach and the environment feels different.

That reputation is your most powerful recruiting and retention tool. And it is built not in the HR strategy or the compensation package, but in the daily choices of the people who lead.

A Challenge to Preceptors

If you are a preceptor, Tier One, Two, Three, or Four, new to the role or years into it, this challenge is for you.

Remember what it felt like.

Not the clinical confidence you have now. The uncertainty you had before it. The shift when you weren't sure, the patient whose presentation surprised you, the moment you reached the edge of what you knew and had to find your way forward without a map.

Your orientee is living that right now. Every shift. In the rooms you walk into together and in the ones they navigate alone after you.

You have something they need that no textbook, no competency checklist, and no mandatory module can provide: the experience of having been where they are and found the way through. The clinical reasoning that has become automatic for you was once effortful and frightening. The confidence you carry was once completely absent. You built it, through experience, through mistakes, through the gradual accumulation of clinical encounters that formed the expert pattern recognition you now use without thinking.

Think out loud. Share the process. Let them hear inside a clinical mind that has been where theirs is going. Not to perform expertise. To transfer it.

And take care of yourself in this role. Attend the Preceptor Power Hours. Use the tools. Ask for what you need. Because a preceptor who feels equipped, seen, and connected is a preceptor who changes trajectories. And a preceptor who is burned out, unsupported, and invisible eventually stops being able to give what their orientee needs.

You are not just a trainer. You are the single most influential person in a new RT's early career. That is not a burden. It is a privilege. Carry it with intention.

A Challenge to the Respiratory Therapy Profession

And now, the largest challenge. The one that goes beyond any individual department, any single educator, or any one book.

The respiratory therapy profession needs to decide what it values.

If it values clinical excellence, and it does, genuinely and demonstrably, then it must be willing to invest in the human infrastructure that produces and sustains clinical excellence. Not just in the equipment, the protocols, and the continuing education credits. In the people. In the development of the educators who develop the clinicians. In the preparation of the preceptors who shape the new graduates. In the careers of the experienced RTs who are one uninvested year away from leaving.

The AARC has the platform. The state societies have the reach. The academic programs have the pipeline. The clinical sites have the relationships. What has been missing is the coordinated, sustained, profession-wide commitment to treating workforce development as the clinical priority it actually is.

Every RT who leaves the profession within two years is a loss that extends beyond the department that couldn't keep them. It is a loss to the patients who will never be cared for by the clinician they might have become. It is a loss to the new graduates who will never be mentored by the experienced RT who burned out before they could give back what they received. It is a loss to the profession's future, a future that depends on the willingness of today's clinicians to invest in tomorrow's.

We can change this. Not with one book. Not with one educator building one department's development program in the margins of an under-resourced role. But with the collective decision made by enough educators, enough leaders, enough preceptors, enough professional organizations, that respiratory therapy is a profession worth investing in. That its people are worth developing. That orientation is the beginning, not the end, of what we owe the clinicians we ask to care for the most vulnerable people in our communities.

That decision starts here. In this book. In the department you walk into tomorrow. In the Preceptor Power Hour that you schedule for next month. In the career conversation you have with the RT who has never been asked where they want to go. In the Clinical Collaboration Summit you invite one academic partner to attend. In the badge you pin on the preceptor who didn't think it was her ministry, and the gospel song you sing when she lets you.

It starts with you. It starts now. It starts Monday.

The Real Measure

I want to end where this book began, not with a framework, a tool, or a data point, but with a person.

The RT who stays five years and preceptors the next new hire.

The one who walks into the orientation of a brand-new graduate, nervous, uncertain, carrying all the hope and all the anxiety of someone who has chosen a profession and is not yet sure it has chosen them back, and says, from experience and from genuine investment: *I've been where you are. Here's what I know. Here's how I think. Here's what I'm going to show you, not just how to do this, but how to think about it.*

That RT, the one who stayed, who grew, who led, and who is now giving back what they were given, is the real measure of this work. Not the retention metric. Not the competency pass rate. Not the survey score or the application number or the conference presentation.

The person.

The clinician who became more than they thought they could be because someone invested in them, and who is now investing in someone else, carrying forward a culture of development that will outlast every program, every initiative, and every book that contributed to building it.

That is what we are building. That is what every Preceptor Power Hour is for. Every Clinical Reasoning Passport. Every Level Up Week. Every badge pinned on a reluctant preceptor who turned out to be extraordinary.

Every career conversation with an RT who had never been asked where they wanted to go. Every check-in with a new graduate who felt dropped off in the middle of nowhere and needed someone to say: you are not alone.

The respiratory therapy profession does not have a clinical problem. It has a development problem. And development problems are human problems, solved not by better equipment or more efficient protocols but by better investment in the people who show up every shift, in every unit, in every hospital across this country, and do the extraordinary, invisible, life-saving work of keeping people breathing.

They deserve better than orientation and silence.

They deserve *Think. Lead. Stay.*

Go build it.

"The respiratory therapy profession does not have a clinical problem. It has a development problem.
And development problems are solved by investing in people."

15

A LETTER TO THE NEW RT

For every respiratory therapist who is just beginning, and for the one you are still becoming.

Dear New RT,

I see you.

Not just the version of you that showed up for orientation with your new badge and your clean scrubs and the particular energy of someone who has worked incredibly hard to get here and is not entirely sure what happens next. I see the version underneath that one, the one that is quietly wondering if they are ready, if they belong here, if the gap between what they learned in school and what this job actually requires is something they will be able to close.

It is. You will. Keep reading.

I want to tell you some things that nobody told me when I was where you are. Things I learned the hard way over twenty years, across multiple states and more clinical settings than I can count on both hands. Things I have watched new RTs need and not receive, and that I have made it my life's work to make sure the next generation (your generation) does not have to figure out alone.

It Is Supposed to Feel Hard

The first thing I want you to know is this: the difficulty you are feeling right now is not evidence that you made the wrong choice. It is evidence that you made a real one.

Respiratory therapy is hard. Not just physically, though the nights are long and the patients are critical and the decisions are high-stakes in ways your training prepared you for intellectually, but nothing fully prepares you for emotionally. It is hard because it asks you to be present (fully, clinically, humanly present) with people at the most frightening moments of their lives. To hold both the technical complexity and the human weight of that simultaneously. To be capable and compassionate at the same time, shift after shift, even on the days when you are tired and uncertain and the patient in front of you is not following the textbook.

That is hard. It is supposed to be hard. And the fact that it feels hard does not mean you are failing. It means you are paying attention. It means you care. And caring, in this profession, is not a liability. It is your greatest clinical asset.

What I Wish Someone Had Told Me

I wish someone had told me that the transition from student to respiratory therapist is one of the most disorienting experiences a professional can go through, and that the disorientation is normal, temporary, and survivable.

You know more than you think you do. And you know less than you will need to know, but that is true of every clinician at every stage of their career, including the ones who look completely certain from the outside. Certainty, in medicine, is almost always a performance. What you are building is something better: genuine clinical reasoning. The ability to sit with uncertainty, work through it systematically, and make the best decision available with the information you have. That takes time. Give yourself the time.

I wish someone had told me that asking for help is not weakness. It is the most clinically responsible thing you can do. The RT who says, "I'm not sure, can you help me think through this?" is protecting their patient. The RT who guesses rather than asks is not. Ask. Every time. Without apology. The colleagues who matter will respect you for it.

I wish someone had told me that your preceptor is human. That they are doing their best with the tools they have, and that sometimes their tools are limited, not because they don't care about your development, but because nobody taught them how to teach. If your preceptor is struggling to explain the why behind the what, it is not a reflection of your inadequacy. It is a gap in their preparation. Find the educator. Find another resource. Keep asking until the why becomes clear.

I wish someone had told me that the hard shifts (the ones where everything went wrong, where the patient didn't make it, where you drove home replaying every decision wondering what you could have done differently), those shifts are not evidence that you don't belong here. They are the shifts that make you the clinician you are becoming. Debrief them. Talk about them. Write about them in your Clinical Reasoning Passport. Let them teach you. And then let them go, because carrying every difficult shift indefinitely is a weight no human being can sustain, and this profession needs you to be sustainable.

What I See in You That You Cannot Yet See in Yourself

You are already leading.

I know you don't believe that. I know that leadership feels like something that belongs to other people (the charge therapist, the supervisor, the one who has been here for ten years and seems to know everything). I know that from where you are standing, the distance between who you are now and who a leader is feels immeasurable.

But listen to me.

Every time you advocate for a patient: when you flag a change in their status before the monitor alarms, when you question an order that doesn't match what you see at the bedside, when you stay five minutes past the end of your shift because something doesn't feel right and you need to make sure the next RT knows, you are leading. Every time you tell a family member, in plain language, what is happening, why, and what you are going to do about it, you are leading. Every time you choose to do the harder right thing instead of the easier wrong one, you are leading.

Leadership is not a title. It is a choice. And you are making it already, shift by shift, decision by decision, through the small, accumulated choices that are forming the clinician, the colleague, and the professional you are becoming.

Own it. You have already started.

What This Profession Will Ask of You

This profession will ask a great deal of you. I want to be honest about that, because the recruiter's version of respiratory therapy and the 3 a.m. version are different experiences, and you deserve to know what you have signed up for.

It will ask you to be technically excellent and emotionally present at the same time. To make high-stakes decisions under pressure with incomplete information. To be the calm in rooms that are anything but. To care deeply about patients you will never see again and colleagues you will see every shift for years. To keep growing when the shift is over and the learning never really is.

It will ask you to advocate: for your patients, for your colleagues, for the profession, and for yourself. To speak up when something is wrong, even when speaking up is uncomfortable. To hold clinical standards high even when the culture around you has let them slip. To be the kind of RT that patients deserve, not just the kind that gets through the shift.

It will eventually ask you to develop someone else. To become the preceptor, the mentor, the experienced colleague who gives back what was given to them. And when that time comes, I hope you will say yes. Not because it is easy. Because it is how the profession survives. Because somewhere right now there is a new RT who will need exactly what you will have to offer, and who will be shaped, in ways that last a career, by whether someone like you showed up for them.

What It Will Give Back

And here is what this profession gives in return.

It gives you purpose that most people spend their whole lives looking for and never find. The knowledge (concrete, specific, undeniable) that what you do changes whether people live or die, breathe or suffocate, recover or deteriorate. That your presence at the bedside, your clinical reasoning, your advocacy, your skill: these things matter in the most fundamental way that anything can matter.

It gives you a community. The particular bond of people who have stood together in the hardest rooms and carried the weight of that together. Colleagues who become friends. Patients who become stories you tell for the rest of your life. Mentors who see something in you before you can see it in yourself, and who, if you are fortunate, you will one day become for someone else.

It gives you a career that keeps growing if you let it. There is no ceiling in respiratory therapy for the clinician who is willing to keep learning. The certifications, the specialties, the leadership roles, the educator pathways, the academic opportunities: the path forward is longer and richer than most people entering this profession realize. You will not exhaust it. Not in twenty years. Not in forty.

And it gives you the moments. The ones that don't make it into the documentation: the hand you held, the family you reassured, the patient who looked at you from across the ventilator circuit with something in their eyes that said, *I know you are trying to save me,* and you were. Those moments are yours. Nobody can take them. And they accumulate, over a career, into something bigger than any single shift or any single patient or any single year. They accumulate into a life's work.

Before You Go

A few last things, from someone who has been doing this for twenty years and is still learning.

Take care of yourself. Not when things slow down, they won't. Now. Rest when you can. Debrief when you need to. Ask for help before the cup is empty. You cannot pour from an empty cup. And this profession needs you full.

Find your people. The colleagues who challenge you, support you, and tell you the truth. They exist in your department and in your professional organizations, and on the other side of a LinkedIn connection with someone doing the same work in a different city. Build that community intentionally. It will sustain you through more than you can currently anticipate.

Get involved. Join your state society. Attend the GSRC meeting, the AARC conference, the regional forums. Not just for the CEUs, though get those too, and not just the ones that are required. Earn more than the minimum. Always. Because the RT who does the minimum required to maintain their license is doing the minimum for their patients too, and you are better than that.

Get the credentials: ACCS, NPS, SDS, AE-C, RPFT, whatever aligns with the population you serve and the clinician you are becoming. Not because letters after your name define your worth, because they don't. But because the pursuit of those credentials forces you to go deeper into the clinical knowledge that makes you genuinely better at the bedside. The studying matters as much as the certification. The process is the point.

Attend the conferences, not just to network, but to learn. To sit in a session and hear someone describe a problem you have been living with and realize you are not alone in it. To present your own work someday, because you have more to contribute to this profession than you currently believe, and the conference room is where that contribution becomes visible. To ask the uncomfortable question in a room full of strangers, the way I once did, and discover that the question you were afraid to ask was the one everyone needed to hear.

Stay connected to the professional community beyond your department. Follow the AARC. Read the journals. Subscribe to the clinical practice guidelines updates. Know what is happening in your field, not just in your unit. The RT who is only as current as their last in-service is not as prepared as the one who is reading, attending, questioning, and growing continuously.

Keep asking why. In the clinical setting. In the professional literature. In the conferences, the courses, and the conversations with colleagues who challenge you. Why does this protocol exist? Why does this patient's response differ from what the research predicts? Why does this department do things this way, and is there a better way? Why have I always done it like this, and is that still the right reason?

The why is where excellence lives. Chase it your whole career. Never stop.

And know this: know it on the hard days especially, when the shift is too long and the decisions are too heavy and you are sitting in your car wondering if you have what it takes:

You were chosen for this.

Not accidentally. Not by default. You chose this profession and it chose you back, in the academic program that trained you, in the department that hired you, in the educator who is reading over your shoulder right now and sees, in you, everything that this profession needs next.

You are already leading. You are already growing. You are already becoming the RT that your next patient needs you to be.

Think deeply. Lead bravely. Stay because the profession needs you, the patients need you, and the new RT who will one day look to you the way you are looking to someone right now needs you to still be here when they arrive.

Think. Lead. Stay.

With everything I have,
The Friendly Educator

"You were chosen for this. Think deeply. Lead bravely. Stay."

www.ingramcontent.com/pod-product-compliance
Ingram Content Group UK Ltd.
Pitfield, Milton Keynes, MK11 3LW, UK
UKHW020200290926
15471UKWH00005B/982

9 798996 349401